Updates in Surgery

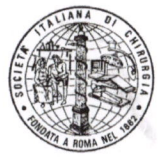

The aim of this series is to provide informative updates on hot topics in the areas of breast, endocrine, and abdominal surgery, surgical oncology, and coloproctology, and on new surgical techniques such as robotic surgery, laparoscopy, and minimally invasive surgery. Readers will find detailed guidance on patient selection, performance of surgical procedures, and avoidance of complications. In addition, a range of other important aspects are covered, from the role of new imaging tools to the use of combined treatments and postoperative care.

The topics addressed by volumes in the series Updates in Surgery have been selected for their broad significance in collaboration with the Italian Society of Surgery. Each volume will assist surgical residents and fellows and practicing surgeons in reaching appropriate treatment decisions and achieving optimal outcomes. The series will also be highly relevant for surgical researchers.

Stefano Bartoli
Francesco Cortese
Massimo Sartelli
Gabriele Sganga
Editors

Infections in Surgery

Prevention and Management

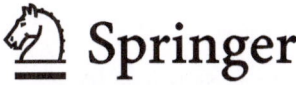 Springer

Editors
Stefano Bartoli
Department of Vascular Surgery
Sant'Eugenio Hospital-ASL Roma 2
Rome, Italy

Francesco Cortese
Emergency Surgery Unit
San Filippo Neri Hospital
Rome, Italy

Massimo Sartelli
Department of Surgery
Macerata Hospital
Macerata, Italy

Gabriele Sganga
Emergency and Trauma Surgery Unit
Policlinico Universitario A. Gemelli IRCCS
Rome, Italy

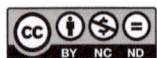

ISSN 2280-9848   ISSN 2281-0854   (electronic)
Updates in Surgery

ISBN 978-3-031-60461-4   ISBN 978-3-031-60462-1   (eBook)
https://doi.org/10.1007/978-3-031-60462-1

The publication and the distribution of this volume have been supported by the Italian Society of Surgery.

The Editors of the volume and the Italian Society of Surgery would like to thank Johnson & Johnson MedTech and Becton, Dickinson Italia S.p.A. for their unconditional contribution, which made it possible to publish this book under the Open Access model.

This book is an open access publication.

Revision and editing: R. M. Martorelli, Scienzaperta (Novate Milanese, Italy)

This Springer imprint is published by the registered company Springer Nature Switzerland AG
The registered company address is: Gewerbestrasse 11, 6330 Cham, Switzerland

If disposing of this product, please recycle the paper.

Foreword

Asepsis, which today is a prerequisite and an integral part of any surgical procedure, even the most trivial, is a practice that we could say has been recently acquired. It was 1847 when Semmelweis intuited, on the basis of empirical observations, that there was a relationship between puerperal fevers and the hygienic conditions of women in labor, but he was isolated and ridiculed by the medical community and died condemned to contempt in the Budapest asylum, as the beautiful biography that Celine dedicated to him tells us. It took another 50 years, and the studies of Louis Pasteur, for the etiological relationship between microorganisms and infectious disease to be demonstrated, but since then the surgeon's field of action has certainly expanded. Asepsis, along with anesthesia, revolutionized the role of surgery in medicine, allowing it to write important chapters in its history. The surgeon's skill could finally save lives without the onset of infections threatening the outcome of the operations.

Therefore, operating in aseptic environments, washing hands and adopting the rules of prophylaxis derived from the maturation and application of Pasteur's studies was to make surgery evolve quickly and achieve extraordinary results in a very short time. This led to the birth and consolidation of the concept of safety of treatments, thanks to which surgery would be able to change the natural course of a disease and truly help to decrease mortality from many diseases by reducing the risk of infections.

The value of surgery today has not changed. On the contrary, it continues to undergo small and large revolutions, and the current minimally invasive techniques with their ability to guarantee conservative approaches constitute the clinician's tool of choice for the treatment of many pathological conditions.

And yet, just over a century later, surgery is still not free from the risk of infection and, due to the increase in the antibiotic resistance, healthcare-associated infections linked to surgical procedures are an incredibly topical and important issue for the health of patients.

Surgical site infections, among the most common of the healthcare-associated infections, are associated with many adverse outcomes causing illness, additional surgical procedures, intensive care unit admissions, and higher mortality.

The scientific literature tells us that about 0.5–3% of patients who undergo surgery will experience an infection at or near the site of surgical incision and that patients who undergo surgery and develop an infection related to surgical care have an average duration of hospitalization that is about 7–11 days longer than those who do not.

This means a threat to health, the economy and, above all, to the sustainability of care.

These figures, however, are not written in stone. Actions can be promoted to reverse this trend and preserve the sustainability of public health protection systems. The World Health Organization states that 40–60% of these infections can be avoided by implementing preventive measures during hospitalization, before and after surgery. To this end, a precise pathway must be followed: the staff need to be educated, trained, and sensitized, and actions must be put in place to improve adherence to counterstrategies against infection.

This book offers numerous knowledge tools and represents an important update for professionals, as well as a valuable aid to promote greater awareness of this phenomenon. In various chapters, both general and specific aspects of the problem are addressed in a detailed and exhaustive way: epidemiology, risk factors, the impact of these infections, as well as the role of measures such as surveillance, antimicrobial stewardship, and Health Technology Assessment.

The contributing authors are all professionals in the field, whose great authority and experience have enabled them to merge clinical skills and expertise in public health, to address the issue with a complete and exhaustive approach. The merit of this volume, therefore, lies not only in having collected and brought up to date the available evidence on infections related to surgical care, but also in having presented and provided, from a public health perspective, the necessary tools to reduce the impact of this scourge that is expensive in economic terms but dramatically more costly in terms of human lives.

September 2024   Rocco Bellantone
Rome, Italy

Foreword

The first Biennial Report of the Italian Society of Surgery was published in 1994, exactly 30 years ago, and in the intervening period infections in surgery have never been addressed, perhaps because surgeons do their work predominantly in the operating room, and most of their concerns are inevitably directed at surgery.

This has led many surgeons to mistakenly consider surgical infections to be a secondary aspect of their practice, but today the surgeon is at the forefront of infection control and management, is responsible for many of the processes that influence infection risk and plays a key role in prophylaxis. Nevertheless, infection prevention, control measures, and some practices, such as proper antibiotic prescription, are often inadequate.

For this reason in recent years, the leading surgical scientific societies have dedicated great attention to this topic, a sign of growing awareness of the problem.

The Italian Society of Surgery is at the front line of this challenge and that is why the Society Governing Council and I enthusiastically welcomed Stefano Bartoli's proposal to publish a monograph on infections in surgery.

The involvement of Francesco Cortese, Massimo Sartelli, and Gabriele Sganga as co-editors and co-authors, and of many experts as co-authors of the 22 chapters forming the book, was Stefano Bartoli's winning choice for writing a work of the highest scientific value. To all of them go my heartfelt thanks for this excellent volume, which addresses all aspects of infections in surgery, from epidemiology to prevention, diagnosis, and treatment, as well as economic and medico-legal implications.

The treatise will surely be a reference for anyone, surgeons and non-surgeons alike, and aspires to be considered a real guideline, which can also be adopted by our Ministry of Health.

September 2024　　　　　　　　　　　　　　　　　　　　　　　Massimo Carlini
Rome, Italy

Preface

Despite proper precautions and intraoperative measures, healthcare-associated infections remain a major concern, increasing overall morbidity and mortality. These infections are acquired by patients receiving medical care and represent the most frequent adverse event affecting patient safety worldwide. The most common healthcare-associated infections include surgical site infections, catheter-associated urinary tract infections, central-line-associated bloodstream infections, hospital-acquired pneumonia, ventilator-associated pneumonia, and *Clostridioides difficile* infection.

While significant progress has been made in infection prevention and control, one of the factors hindering the prevention of infections in surgery is the uneven implementation of recommended prevention practices due to low awareness of the problem, which is often viewed as episodic and not related to systemic factors. Hospital-acquired infections reflect an organizational deviation from best practices that recommend adequate assessment of the patient's characteristics and of the hospital environment.

Preventing infections in surgery requires a multidisciplinary and multiprofessional approach. Adherence to guidelines and protocols, early recognition and proper treatment are key to significantly reducing infection rates and improving surgical outcomes.

Through the contribution of many experts from different disciplines, this book aims to provide surgeons with a useful tool to further their understanding of the various aspects of surgical infections, including prevention and control of infections and potential sources, antimicrobial stewardship, and management of sepsis. In each chapter, the reader will be able to find, thanks to the authors' experience, practical suggestions to tackle the problem of infections in surgery.

Thanks to the unconditional contribution of Johnson & Johnson MedTech and Becton, Dickinson Italia S.p.A., the book is made available as open access so as to reach a broad readership.

September 2024
Rome, Italy   Stefano Bartoli
Rome, Italy   Francesco Cortese
Macerata, Italy   Massimo Sartelli
Rome, Italy   Gabriele Sganga

Contents

Guidelines and Good Clinical Practice in Surgical Infection

1

Stefano Bartoli, Giulia Ianni, Gianluca Smedile, Tommaso Castrucci, and Andrea Siani

1.1 Introduction

Despite proper precautions and intraoperative measures, healthcare-associated infections (HAIs) remain a major concern, increasing overall morbidity and mortality, with an incidence similar to hospital-acquired pneumonia or urinary tract infections. These are acquired by patients while receiving medical care and represent the most frequent adverse event that negatively impacts patient safety worldwide.

Surgical incision and some medical devices such as central lines, urinary catheters and ventilators, seem to be contributing factors leading to the development of HAIs [1, 2]. Surgical site infections (SSIs) are the most common HAIs and continue to be a major clinical problem in terms of morbidity and mortality, length of hospital stay, and financial cost. The World Health Organization (WHO) [3, 4] and the Centers for Disease Control and Prevention (CDC) [5] have published guidelines for the prevention of SSIs. Knowledge of infection prevention and control (IPC) seems to be central in preventing SSIs and avoiding inadequate approaches.

An SSI is a HAI in which a wound becomes infected after an invasive, generally surgical, procedure. The most common HAIs include SSIs, catheter-associated urinary tract infections (CAUTIs), central-line-associated bloodstream infections (CLABSIs), hospital-acquired pneumonia (HAP), ventilator-associated pneumonia (VAP), and *Clostridioides difficile* infection.

S. Bartoli (✉) · G. Ianni · G. Smedile · T. Castrucci · A. Siani
Department of Vascular Surgery, Sant'Eugenio Hospital-ASL Roma 2, Rome, Italy
e-mail: steba08@gmail.com; giuliaianni@hotmail.com; gianlucasmedile69@gmail.com; tcastrucci@gmail.com; andreasiani@yahoo.it

© The Author(s) 2025
S. Bartoli et al. (eds.), *Infections in Surgery*, Updates in Surgery,
https://doi.org/10.1007/978-3-031-60462-1_1

SSIs represent 20% of all HAIs, and 5% of patients undergoing a surgical procedure develop an SSI. Moreover, the incidence of SSI is conditioned by the increasingly aging population, obesity, immunodepression, diabetes and increasingly complex procedures. In addition, growing numbers of infections are now being seen in primary care because patients are discharged earlier in fast-track surgery [3, 6].

The most frequently identified bacteria include Gram-positive microorganisms, such as *Staphylococcus aureus*, coagulase-negative Staphylococci, *Enterococcus* spp., and *Escherichia coli*. Gram-negative bacteria including Enterobacterales may also cause SSIs, especially after abdominal procedures.

Antibiotic resistance, HAIs, and IPC are interrelated aspects; many HAIs are in fact caused by antibiotic-resistant germs and are associated with significant increases in the length of hospitalization and costs [7]. The main factors that drive antibiotic resistance and cause its problems are the improper use and abuse of antimicrobials in the human and veterinary field and HAIs especially in the surgical field [8].

1.2 Good Practice and Global Guidelines for the Prevention of Surgical Site Infections

An SSI ranges from limited wound infection to a life-threatening postoperative complication and is generally caused by contamination of the incision site with the patient's own body microorganisms during surgery. SSIs can have a significant effect on the patients' quality of life, increasing morbidity and length of hospital stay, with an important financial burden for healthcare providers. To reduce the risk of infection, some measures can be put in place during the pre-, intra-, and postoperative care phases. For example, a correct postoperative management of surgical wounds can reduce the rate of SSIs, although patient-related risk factors, type of surgery and surgical technique are parts of a more general evaluation process (Chaps. 15 and 16).

The guideline recommendations for prevention and management of SSI are based on rigorous evaluation of the best available published evidence (strong or conditional). Currently, the 2016 WHO global guidelines include recommendations for the preoperative period to prevent the infections during and after surgical procedures: for example, showering before surgery, appropriate disinfection of the surgical team, correct use of prophylactic antibiotics, and type of operation site disinfectants and sutures to be used. The guidelines recommend antibiotic prophylaxis (ABP) to prevent infections only before and during surgery without evidence supporting postoperative ABP. Indeed, in contrast to consolidated habits among surgeons, antibiotics should not be used after surgery. Usually, ABP should be administered only in surgical procedures at high risk for SSI or when foreign materials are implanted. ABP should be administered within 120 min prior to the incision or based on its pharmacological proprieties.

Some underlying patient features may affect drug pharmacokinetics such as malnourishment, obesity, cachexia, or renal disease (protein loss led to suboptimal antibiotic exposure through increased antibiotic clearance in the presence of normal or augmented renal function). Additional antibiotic doses should be administered intraoperatively for procedures lasting >2–4 h (typically where duration exceeds two half-lives of the antibiotic) (Chaps. 7 and 8).

The surgical preoperative and intraoperative checklist can help to improve patient outcomes regarding SSIs and the occurrence of intraoperative errors.

1.3 Improving Infection Prevention and Control

Many HAIs may be prevented, and several measures can reduce the risk of HAIs: hence, the emphasis on the need for a team of operators who act in unison following evidence-based recommendations and discouraging individual initiatives not supported by evidence. Data analysis and control of all those maneuvers aimed at reducing infections are fundamental, as is attention to valorizing human resources to obtain the common good (Chaps. 2 and 4).

Attention is paid not only to the purely clinical impact of infections, which is different in the various types of surgery, but also to the broader and more extensive aspect of costs at a national and global level (Chaps. 3, 20, 22).

According to a meta-analysis of studies evaluating the results of diverse interventions to reduce HAIs in acute care or long-term care settings by Schreiber et al. [9], HAI incidence can be reduced to the range of 35–55% by means of multifaceted interventions. An IPC program is essential in each hospital to coordinate the education and training of professional workers according to evidence-based guidelines and supporting the surveillance and monitoring of HAIs through implementation of multimodal strategies, as recommended by the WHO. The expression "multimodal strategy" should be understood as the use of multiple approaches that can influence the behavior of healthcare workers, impacting patient outcomes and contributing to organizational change.

A significant portion of HAI can be prevented by adopting evidence-based care practices. Interventions that use a multimodal approach are effective in preventing infections by breaking down obstacles relating to individual professionals and the social, organizational and economic contexts (Chaps. 4–6).

Currently, several tools to transfer best practices into routine clinical care and to support guideline implementation are available, including "care bundles". Bundles are simple sets of evidence-based IPC measures that can improve both patient outcomes and the "culture" of patient safety. Bundles used as stand-alone interventions or as part of multimodal strategies have been widely associated with decreased rates of CLABSI, VAP, SSIs, and CAUTIs, as reported by Sartelli et al. in 2023 [10]. The components to be included in prevention bundles are suggested in Table 1.1. Surgical checklists are a simple strategy for addressing surgical patient safety. They can potentially prevent errors from occurring during or after surgery. Although there is no great evidence in the literature, checklists have largely been considered important tools (Chaps. 9, 10, 14).

Table 1.1 Prevention bundles for healthcare-associated infections

HAI	Components of the prevention bundles
CLABSI	*Insertion bundle*: – Maintaining maximal sterile barrier precautions – Cleaning the skin with alcohol-based chlorhexidine – Avoiding the femoral vein for central line insertion in adult patients – Having dedicated staff for central line insertion – Having available insertion guidelines (including indications for central line use) and use of checklists with trained observers *Maintenance bundle*: – Evaluating central line necessity daily – Removing unnecessary lines promptly – Disinfecting before manipulation of the line
CAUTI	*Insertion bundle*: – Avoiding the use of urinary catheters if not necessary – Using a correct insertion technique to minimize contamination *Maintenance bundle*: – Maintaining a closed drainage system to avoid catheter colonization – Assessing the daily need for indwelling urinary catheters – Avoiding routine antimicrobial prophylaxis in patients with a urinary catheter
VAP	*Maintenance bundle*: – Elevating the head of the bed to between 30 and 45 degrees – Assessing daily readiness to extubate the patient – Performing daily oral care with chlorhexidine – Stopping unnecessary proton pump inhibitors – Using subglottic secretion drainage
SSI	*PAP administration bundle*: – Administering appropriate PAP – Administering PAP within 120 min before the incision according to the pharmacokinetic profiles of the antibiotic – Redosing the antibiotic for prolonged procedures (where duration exceeds two half-lives of the antibiotic) and in patients with major blood loss (>1.5 L) – Discontinuing antibiotics after surgery *Perioperative measures bundle*: – Avoiding hair removal and, if necessary, using electric clippers – Using alcohol-based disinfectant for surgical site preparation – Maintaining intraoperative glycemic control with target blood glucose levels <200 mg/dL – Maintaining perioperative normothermia with a target temperature >36 °C

HAI healthcare-associated infection, *CLABSI* central-line-associated bloodstream infection, *CAUTI* catheter-associated urinary tract infection, *VAP* ventilator-associated pneumonia, *SSI* surgical site infection, *PAP* perioperative antibiotic prophylaxis

1.4 Improving Healthcare in Surgical Site Infection Prevention and Control

Despite SSI prevention strategies having been defined, their application in routine daily practice seems to be uniformly poor due to intrapersonal, interpersonal and institutional/organizational factors. Regarding the intra- and interpersonal factors, increasing knowledge and skills alone may not be sufficient to effect sustained change especially considering the multifactorial nature of HAIs. Indeed, the acquisition of new behavioral attitudes and norms based on clinical evidence and not on previous experience may positively influence SSI prevention and control. The creation of a multidisciplinary task force within the hospital is mandatory to manage the problem and to allow strategies and solutions. This can mobilize the hospital resources in the direction of implementing strategies, promoting collaboration, coordination, communication, teamwork and efficient patient care organization [11].

Patient-related factors are also important. Attention to some fields of surgery, such as prosthetic, vascular, orthopedic or abdominal surgery (Chaps. 11–14), and to particular classes of patients, such as immunocompromised patients, is fundamental not only for prophylaxis but also for the epidemiology, microbiology and treatment of infections which require special care both immediately, with a highly personalized approach, and in the postoperative period, which often occurs in intensive care units (Chaps. 17–19).

Multidisciplinary teams have been shown to be clinically effective both in improving patient outcomes and in reducing costs: hence, the focus on source control (SC), i.e., interventions aimed at identifying and eliminating (or controlling) the source of infection to restore normal homeostasis. Combined with targeted antibiotic therapy, SC is essential in the management of intra-abdominal and other infections, thus becoming part of a multidisciplinary and multimodal approach rather than an exclusively surgical one (Chap. 14). In the context of postoperative patient management, Enhanced Recovery After Surgery (ERAS) protocols, applied in different specialties, show a reduction in the length of hospital stay, complication rates and costs compared to traditional perioperative care even though their role in reducing postoperative infections is still unclear. Integration of the ERAS program and preventive care can lead to a cumulative and synergistic effect to reduce the likelihood of developing postoperative infections (Chap. 18).

The legal implication of infections should not be overlooked; the possibility of medical liability arising from HAIs has brought to light over the years the high level of complexity of ascertaining causal links. From a medicolegal point of view, the difficulty in ascertaining the events directly leading to the infectious incident resides in the variability of the causes. The expert must first ascertain whether the infection is directly attributable to the healthcare facility or to the conduct of the healthcare personnel (fault or negligence) (Chap. 21).

1.5 Conclusion

The occurrence of HAIs remains a problem with increasing incidence. Guidelines for the prevention of SSIs suggest that healthcare workers should develop an evidence-based program to implement IPC with a focus on surgical safety as well as antimicrobial resistance action plans. Multimodal intervention strategies, based on behavioral theories and reported experiences, seem to be more effective than personal or less team-directed approaches.

References

1. Haque M, Sartelli M, McKimm J, Abu BM. Health care-associated infections—an overview. Infect Drug Resist. 2018;11:2321–33.
2. Sartelli M, Pagani L, Iannazzo S, et al. A proposal for a comprehensive approach to infections across the surgical pathway. World J Emerg Surg. 2020;15(1):13.
3. World Health Organization. Global action plan on antimicrobial resistance. Geneva: WHO; 2015. https://www.who.int/publications/i/item/9789241509763. Accessed 16 Mar 2024.
4. European Centre for Disease Prevention and Control. Assessing the health burden of infections with antibiotic-resistant bacteria in the EU/EEA, 2016–2020. Stockholm: ECDC; 2022. https://www.ecdc.europa.eu/en/publications-data/health-burden-infections-antibiotic-resistant-bacteria-2016-2020. Accessed 16 Mar 2024.
5. Berríos-Torres SI, Umscheid CA, Bratzler DW, et al. Centers for Disease Control and Prevention guideline for the prevention of surgical site infection, 2017. JAMA Surg. 2017;152(8):784–91. Erratum in: JAMA Surg. 2017;152(8):803.
6. Allegranzi B, Bischoff P, de Jonge S, et al. New WHO recommendations on preoperative measures for surgical site infection prevention: an evidence based global perspective. Lancet Infect Dis. 2016;16(12):e276–87.
7. Sartelli M, Coccolini F, Abu-Zidan FM, et al. Hey surgeons! It is time to lead and be a champion in preventing and managing surgical infections! World J Emerg Surg. 2020;15(1):28.
8. Holmes AH, Moore LS, Sundsfjord A, et al. Understanding the mechanisms and drivers of antimicrobial resistance. Lancet. 2016;387(10014):176–87.
9. Schreiber PW, Sax H, Wolfensberger A, et al. The preventable proportion of healthcare-associated infections 2005–2016: systematic review and meta-analysis. Infect Control Hosp Epidemiol. 2018;39(11):1277–95.
10. Sartelli M, Bartoli S, Borghi F, et al. Implementation strategies for preventing healthcare-associated infections across the surgical pathway: an Italian multisociety document. Antibiotics (Basel). 2023;12(3):521.
11. Sartelli M, Kluger Y, Ansaloni L, et al. Knowledge, awareness, and attitude towards infection prevention and management among surgeons: identifying the surgeon champion. World J Emerg Surg. 2018;13:37.

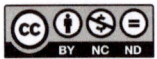

Impact of Healthcare-Associated Infections in Surgery

2

Fortunato "Paolo" D'Ancona and Claudia Isonne

2.1 Introduction

Healthcare-associated infections (HAIs) are acquired by patients while receiving care and represent the most frequent adverse event affecting the patient's safety worldwide. These infections are often caused by microorganisms resistant to commonly used antimicrobials and are usually multidrug-resistant [1, 2]. They have a dramatic impact on physical, mental/emotional, and financial health [3].

It is estimated that across the European Union/European Economic Area (EU/EEA) countries the burden of HAIs in 2011–2012 was almost twice the burden of other 32 infections in terms of disability and premature mortality [4, 5]. It is estimated that, out of every 100 patients in acute-care hospitals, 7 of them in high-income countries (HICs) and 15 in low- and middle-income countries (LMICs) could acquire at least one HAI during their hospitalization [1, 6].

The European Centre for Disease Prevention and Control (ECDC) reports an HAI prevalence in Europe in 2016–2017 of 5.9% (country range: 2.9–10.0%) [7]; similarly, in the United States (USA), the Centers for Diseases Control (CDC) report an HAI prevalence of 3.2% for 2015 [8], and a survey in the Middle East reported an HAI prevalence of 11.2% [9]. The ECDC estimated that 3.8 million HAIs occur yearly in patients admitted to acute-care hospitals in EU and EEA countries [7]. There is an association between HAI and risk of death: a study in the USA in 2002 reported that 5.8% of the study population that experienced an HAI had a fatal outcome, while in the EU and EEA a model based on 2011 data estimated that 3.5% of the patients with an HAI died [4]. A meta-analysis in 2020 reported that the pooled risk of death increases notably if the HAI is a sepsis (24%); the mortality in

F. "P". D'Ancona (✉) · C. Isonne
Department of Infectious Diseases, Istituto Superiore di Sanità, Rome, Italy
e-mail: paolo.dancona@iss.it; claudia.isonne@iss.it

© The Author(s) 2025
S. Bartoli et al. (eds.), *Infections in Surgery*, Updates in Surgery,
https://doi.org/10.1007/978-3-031-60462-1_2

intensive care units (ICU) was 44.8% for ICU-acquired sepsis and 56.5% in cases of hospital-acquired sepsis with organ dysfunction [10].

2.2   Frequency of Surgical Site Infection

Surgical site infection (SSI) is one of the most frequently reported types of HAI: the ECDC reports that SSIs are up to 18.4% of all HAIs in Europe in 2016–2017 [11]. SSI is the most frequently reported HAI in LMICs [1], but it is actually the most frequent HAI also in some HICs (e.g., Australia [12], Austria, Finland, Norway, the Netherlands [11]). The CDC and ECDC define SSI as a postoperative infection occurring within 30 days of a surgical procedure (or within 1 year for permanent implants) [13].

Overall, data from the ECDC report for 2018–2020 showed a total of 19,680 SSIs in Europe. Among these, 8560 (42%) were classified as superficial SSIs, 6042 (30%) as deep SSIs, and 5720 (28%) as organ/space SSIs. The proportion of deep or organ/space SSIs ranged from 27.0% for cesarean section to 81.0% for hip prosthesis surgery. Out of all SSIs, 30% were diagnosed during the hospital stay, while 50% were detected after discharge [13].

Based on data from the USA, SSI accounts for 20% of all HAIs and is linked to a significant increase in the risk of mortality, ranging from 2 to 11 times higher [14, 15]. Approximately 75% of deaths associated with SSI can be directly attributed to the infection itself.

Crucial patient-related factors that contribute to SSI include pre-existing infections, low levels of serum albumin, advanced age, obesity, smoking, diabetes mellitus, and ischemia resulting from vascular disease or radiation therapy. Surgical risk factors include lengthy procedures and deficiencies in either the surgical scrub or the antiseptic preparation of the skin. Physiological conditions that increase the likelihood of SSI encompass trauma, shock, blood transfusion, hypothermia, hypoxia, and hyperglycemia [2].

The prevalence of SSIs exhibited significant variation depending on the type of surgical procedure. For instance, knee prosthesis surgical operations had a low SSI rate of 0.6%, whereas open colon operations had a higher rate of 9.5%. Additionally, the incidence density of in-hospital SSIs also differed significantly across different types of surgical procedures. In comparison to open procedures, laparoscopic procedures in both cholecystectomy and colon surgery demonstrated lower percentages of SSIs and incidence density. HAIs are also frequently observed following cardiac surgery, with reported incidence rates ranging from 5.0% to 21.7%. These infections are often accompanied by multiple organ failure, prolonged hospital stays, and elevated mortality rates [16]. The condition of the patients may increase the risk of infection: in a recent study of patients with hip fracture, subjects with moderate and severe comorbidity, compared to no comorbidity, had an adjusted hazard ratio of 1.3 and 1.6 of SSI within 0–30 days of surgery, including the increased frequency of reoperation [17].

2.3   Consequences of Surgical Site Infection

The financial burden of SSI is due to the extended hospitalization of the patient, delayed recovery, supplementary diagnostic tests, treatment, reoperation, readmission, transient or permanent loss of function in the affected region, and death [18, 19]. A 2009 review reported that in European hospitals patients with an SSI cost approximately twice the amount of patients who do not develop an SSI and more than double the length of hospitalization [20], without considering the cost for continuing treatment in community settings.

A 2011 review highlighted differences among the study methods used to estimate the costs of SSI, reporting unadjusted mean or median costs per infection falling in the range of 5600–12,900 USD [21]. SSI is considered the most expensive type of HAI, with an estimated annual cost of 3.3 billion USD. Moreover, it prolongs hospital stays by an average of 9.7 days, leading to an additional cost of over 20,000 USD per admission [14, 22].

In 2017, Badia et al. evaluated the evidence for the cost and health-related quality of life (HRQoL) burden of SSI across various surgical specialties in six European countries; in all six countries, SSIs were constantly associated with more elevated costs compared to uninfected patients; however, due to the considerable heterogeneity between the studies, a meta-analysis was not deemed appropriate by the authors [18]. For example, in cardiothoracic surgery, where there is a higher number of studies among the countries, a study conducted in France reported that the total additional cost of an SSI over 4 years for 94 patients was 291,000 and 1,034,000 EUR with and without reimbursement, respectively, and the mean length of stay (LOS) was 23 days in patients with an SSI compared to 10 days in patients without SSI; a higher percentage of patients died during the study period in the first group (5.4% vs. 2.4%) [18]. Similarly, in Germany a significantly higher cost per patient was reported for those who contracted an SSI in comparison to uninfected patients (36,261 and 13,356 EUR respectively, $p < 0.0001$). Furthermore, both the LOS in hospital and the mortality during the 27-month study were significantly higher among infected versus uninfected patients (LOS in hospital, 34.4 vs. 16.5; mortality, 17.6% vs. 8.8%) [18].

In 2020 a systematic review of the economic burden of SSI reported that the range of additional costs of SSI was similar in LMIC (174–29,610 USD) and European countries (21–34,000 USD) [23].

The impact also differs according to the type of surgery: it has been estimated that between 2% and 36% of patients may develop SSIs. Orthopedic surgery was considered the specialty with the highest risk for SSI [18]; in a study evaluating infections in tibial fractures in a Spanish cohort, 17.2% of patients developed SSI with higher hospital LOS (34.9 vs. 12.0 days), more readmissions (1.21 vs. 0.25) and longer mean operating theatre time (499 vs. 219 min). Total in-hospital costs for patients with infection increased from 7607 to 17,538 EUR [24]. In a Danish study of patients with open tibial fractures treated with a free flap, the presence of an SSI increased mean LOS from 28 to 63.8 days, and mean treatment costs from 49,301 to 67,958 EUR [25]. In England, a retrospective study of patients with and without infection following intramedullary nailing for a tibial shaft fracture showed significant increases in in-hospital costs (80%), LOS (109% increase at 1 year), readmissions (5.18 times at 1 year), and reoperations associated with infection (2.47 times at 1 year) [26]. In the Italian context, a model assessed the direct costs of seven SSIs developed following arthroplasty procedures and found that the additional medical costs for SSI relative to uninfected patients were 32,000 EUR, corresponding to an average cost per SSI of 9560 EUR [27].

In the area of gynecologic oncology, data from 2 years of activity of a large Italian center on 5682 patients showed that 322 (5.6%) had an HAI and 248 (77.3%) had undergone surgery (including laparotomy, laparoscopy, bowel resection, bladder resection) in the previous 30 days, with a LOS of 17 days for medical patients and 20 days for surgical patients; on multivariate analysis, advanced age (odds ratio [OR] 1.23), bowel resection (OR 2.66), SSI (OR 10.45), and central venous catheter infection (OR 9.86) were found to be independently associated with prolonged hospital stay (>20 days) [28]. In this cohort, the overall direct cost of HAIs was 6,273,852 USD (mean for each patient 19,484 USD).

A retrospective observational cohort study in Canada between 2011 and 2014 reported that, among patients with liver transplantation, 36 recipients developed SSIs (36/229, 15.7%), with a median LOS of 12 days (IQR 9–21) vs. 10.5 days (IQR 8–20) in recipients without an SSI, with a median LOS cost of 39,456 Canadian dollars and 31,084 Canadian dollars, respectively; the transfusion of ≥5 units of red cells and dialysis before transplantation were reported to be statistically related with higher cost [29].

In European countries, 14.0–22.2% of SSIs are due to abdominal surgery; laparoscopic procedures in both cholecystectomy and colon operations had lower percentages of SSIs and incidence density than open procedures, and the percentage of SSIs per 100 operations amounts to 9.5% in open colon surgery [13]. In a Japanese study, the incidence of SSIs was 11.3% after gastrectomy, 15.5% after colorectal surgery, 11.3% after hepatectomy, and 36.9% after pancreaticoduodenectomy [30].

HAIs are a common postoperative complication also for some specialist oncologic surgeries such as head and neck free-flap reconstruction. In a 2019–2020 Spanish study, 40/65 patients (61.54%) suffered HAIs (SSIs: 52.18%; nosocomial pneumonia: 23.20%; bloodstream infection: 13%; urinary tract infection: 5.80%). The HAIs caused a need to reoperate (OR 6.89), prolonged LOS (OR 1.16) and delay in the initiation of postoperative radiotherapy (OR 9.07). The impact was also evident in the 6-month mortality rate: 7.69% in patients with HAIs vs. 0% in patients without HAIs [31].

SSIs also negatively impact the patients' mental health, partially as a result of pain and anxiety. A study that enrolled 760 patients from 21 centers in the UK measured, as a secondary outcome, HRQoL (using the EuroQoL tool), finding an 11% reduction in HRQoL at 30 days in patients who developed an infection ($p < 0.001$) [32]. Patients experience a notable increase in pain attributed to the infection, leading to a deterioration in their physical function, as well as feelings of insecurity, depression and a sense of unease when observing their wound owing to lack of familiarity with the appearance of a typical healing wound. Patients also reported experiencing mental anguish due to feelings of depression stemming from the long-lasting nature of the infection. Some patients with SSI reported that depression led to social isolation and that the signs and symptoms of the SSI gave rise to feelings of fear and anxiety. There is also a social effect on patients' everyday life, with repercussions for their social network and family relationships [33].

2.4 Conclusion

In conclusion, estimating the frequency, the burden and the additional cost burden caused by the complications of surgery (e.g., an SSI) helps to understand how important it is to reduce HAI and prioritize interventions [34–37]. However, this may prove challenging because SSIs are not always manifest during the hospitalization, the postdischarge monitoring methods may be different [38, 39], the follow-up is not always easy especially in LMICs [40], and the very definition of SSI may differ among countries or studies [41].

References

1. Allegranzi B, Bagheri Nejad S, Combescure C, et al. Burden of endemic health-care-associated infection in developing countries: systematic review and meta-analysis. Lancet. 2011;377(9761):228–41.
2. Cheadle WG. Risk factors for surgical site infection. Surg Infect (Larchmt). 2006;7(Suppl 1):S7–S11.
3. World Health Organization. Global report on infection prevention and control. Geneva: WHO; 2022. https://www.who.int/publications/i/item/9789240051164. Accessed 16 Mar 2024.
4. Cassini A, Plachouras D, Eckmanns T, et al. Burden of six healthcare-associated infections on European population health: estimating incidence-based disability-adjusted life years through a population prevalence-based modelling study. PLoS Med. 2016;13(10):e1002150.
5. Cassini A, Colzani E, Pini A, et al. Impact of infectious diseases on population health using incidence-based disability-adjusted life years (DALYs): results from the Burden of Communicable Diseases in Europe study, European Union and European Economic Area countries, 2009 to 2013. Euro Surveill. 2018;23(16):17-00454.
6. World Health Organization. Report on the burden of endemic health care-associated infection worldwide. Geneva: WHO; 2011. https://www.who.int/publications/i/item/report-on-the-burden-of-endemic-health-care-associated-infection-worldwide. Accessed 16 Mar 2024.
7. Suetens C, Latour K, Kärki T, et al. Prevalence of healthcare-associated infections, estimated incidence and composite antimicrobial resistance index in acute care hospitals and long-term care facilities: results from two European point prevalence surveys, 2016 to 2017. Euro Surveill. 2018;23(46):1800516. Erratum in: Euro Surveill. 2018;23(47):181122e1.
8. Magill SS, O'Leary E, Janelle SJ, et al. Changes in prevalence of health care-associated infections in U.S. hospitals. N Engl J Med. 2018;379(18):1732–44.
9. Alothman A, Al Thaqafi A, Al Ansary A, et al. Prevalence of infections and antimicrobial use in the acute-care hospital setting in the Middle East: results from the first point-prevalence survey in the region. Int J Infect Dis. 2020;101:249–58.
10. Markwart R, Saito H, Harder T, et al. Epidemiology and burden of sepsis acquired in hospitals and intensive care units: a systematic review and meta-analysis. Intensive Care Med. 2020;46(8):1536–51.

11. European Centre for Disease Prevention and Control. Point prevalence survey of healthcare-associated infections and antimicrobial use in European acute care hospitals, 2016–2017. Stockholm: ECDC; 2023. https://www.ecdc.europa.eu/en/publications-data/point-prevalence-survey-healthcare-associated-infections-and-antimicrobial-use-5. Accessed 16 Mar 2024.

12. Lydeamore MJ, Mitchell BG, Bucknall T, et al. Burden of five healthcare associated infections in Australia. Antimicrob Resist Infect Control. 2022;11(1):69. Erratum in: Antimicrob Resist Infect Control. 2022;11(1):129.

13. European Centre for Disease Prevention and Control. Healthcare-associated infections: surgical site infections. In: ECDC. Annual epidemiological report for 2018–2020. Stockholm: ECDC; 2023. https://www.ecdc.europa.eu/en/publications-data/healthcare-associated-infections-surgical-site-annual-2018-2020. Accessed 16 Mar 2024.

14. Ban KA, Minei JP, Laronga C, et al. American College of Surgeons and Surgical Infection Society: surgical site infection guidelines, 2016 update. J Am Coll Surg. 2017;224(1):59–74.

15. Awad SS. Adherence to surgical care improvement project measures and post-operative surgical site infections. Surg Infect (Larchmt). 2012;13(4):234–7.

16. Haque M, Sartelli M, McKimm J, Abu BM. Health care-associated infections—an overview. Infect Drug Resist. 2018;11:2321–33.

17. Gadgaard NR, Varnum C, Nelissen RG, et al. Comorbidity and risk of infection among patients with hip fracture: a Danish population-based cohort study. Osteoporos Int. 2023;34(10):1739–49.

18. Badia JM, Casey AL, Petrosillo N, et al. Impact of surgical site infection on healthcare costs and patient outcomes: a systematic review in six European countries. J Hosp Infect. 2017;96(1):1–15.

19. Cai Y, Lo JJ, Venkatachalam I, et al. The impact of healthcare associated infections on mortality and length of stay in Singapore—a time-varying analysis. Infect Control Hosp Epidemiol. 2020;41(11):1315–20.

20. Broex EC, van Asselt AD, Bruggeman CA, van Tiel FH. Surgical site infections: how high are the costs? J Hosp Infect. 2009;72(3):193–201.

21. Umscheid CA, Mitchell MD, Doshi JA, et al. Estimating the proportion of healthcare-associated infections that are reasonably preventable and the related mortality and costs. Infect Control Hosp Epidemiol. 2011;32(2):101–14.

22. Zimlichman E, Henderson D, Tamir O, et al. Health care-associated infections: a meta-analysis of costs and financial impact on the US health care system. JAMA Intern Med. 2013;173(22):2039–46.

23. Monahan M, Jowett S, Pinkney T, et al. Surgical site infection and costs in low- and middle-income countries: a systematic review of the economic burden. PLoS One. 2020;15(6):e0232960.

24. Barrés-Carsí M, Navarrete-Dualde J, Quintana Plaza J, et al. Healthcare resource use and costs related to surgical infections of tibial fractures in a Spanish cohort. PLoS One. 2022;17(11):e0277482.

25. Olesen UK, Pedersen NJ, Eckardt H, et al. The cost of infection in severe open tibial fractures treated with a free flap. Int Orthop. 2017;41(5):1049–55.

26. Galvain T, Chitnis A, Paparouni K, et al. The economic burden of infections following intra-medullary nailing for a tibial shaft fracture in England. BMJ Open. 2020;10(8):e035404.

27. Nobile M, Navone P, Orzella A, et al. Developing a model for analysis the extra costs associated with surgical site infections (SSIs): an orthopaedic and traumatological study run by the Gaetano Pini Orthopaedic Institute. Antimicrob Resist Infect Control. 2015;4(Suppl 1):P68.

28. Biscione A, Corrado G, Quagliozzi L, et al. Healthcare associated infections in gynecologic oncology: clinical and economic impact. Int J Gynecol Cancer. 2023;33(2):278–84.

29. Natori Y, Vu J, Chow E, et al. The economic impact of increased length of stay associated with surgical site infections in liver transplantation on Canadian healthcare costs. Clin Transpl. 2021;35(1):e14155.

30. Maehara Y, Shirabe K, Kohnoe S, et al. Impact of intra-abdominal absorbable sutures on surgical site infection in gastrointestinal and hepato-biliary-pancreatic surgery: results of a

multicenter, randomized, prospective, phase II clinical trial. Surg Today. 2017;47(9):1060–71. Erratum in: Surg Today. 2017;47(12):1539–40.

31. Ramos-Zayas A, Lopez-Medrano F, Urquiza-Fornovi I, et al. The impact of healthcare-associated infections in patients undergoing oncological microvascular head and neck reconstruction: a prospective multicentre study. Cancers (Basel). 2021;13(9):2109.

32. Pinkney TD, Calvert M, Bartlett DC, et al. Impact of wound edge protection devices on surgical site infection after laparotomy: multicentre randomised controlled trial (ROSSINI trial). BMJ. 2013;347:f4305.

33. Avsar P, Patton D, Ousey K, et al. The impact of surgical site infection on health-related quality of life: a systematic review. Wound Manag Prev. 2021;67(6):10–9.

34. Calderwood MS, Anderson DJ, Bratzler DW, et al. Strategies to prevent surgical site infections in acute-care hospitals: 2022 update. Infect Control Hosp Epidemiol. 2023;44(5):695–720.

35. World Health Organization. Global guidelines for the prevention of surgical site infection. 2nd ed. Geneva: WHO; 2018. https://www.who.int/publications/i/item/9789241550475. Accessed 16 Mar 2024.

36. Berríos-Torres SI, Umscheid CA, Bratzler DW, et al. Centers for Disease Control and Prevention guideline for the prevention of surgical site infection, 2017. JAMA Surg. 2017;152(8):784–91. Erratum in: JAMA Surg. 2017;152(8):803.

37. Tarricone R. Cost-of-illness analysis. What room in health economics? Health Policy. 2006;77(1):51–63.

38. Leaper D, Tanner J, Kiernan M. Surveillance of surgical site infection: more accurate definitions and intensive recording needed. J Hosp Infect. 2013;83(2):83–6.

39. Koek MB, Wille JC, Isken MR, et al. Post-discharge surveillance (PDS) for surgical site infections: a good method is more important than a long duration. Euro Surveill. 2015;20(8):21042.

40. Young S, Lie SA, Hallan G, et al. Low infection rates after 34,361 intramedullary nail operations in 55 low- and middle-income countries: validation of the Surgical Implant Generation Network (SIGN) online surgical database. Acta Orthop. 2011;82(6):737–43.

41. Ashby E, Haddad FS, O'Donnell E, Wilson AP. How will surgical site infection be measured to ensure "high quality care for all"? J Bone Joint Surg Br. 2010;92(9):1294–9.

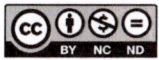

Epidemiological Framework: The Role of Surveillance

3

Enrico Ricchizzi

3.1 Introduction

The systematic collection, analysis, interpretation of data related to surgical procedures, patients, and surgical site infections (SSIs), and the dissemination of the results to surgeons, other members of the surgical teams, and hospital administrators form the process known as *surveillance*.

3.1.1 Aims of Surveillance

Surveillance is one of the essential and indispensable components of an effective infection prevention and control program [1] whose ultimate aim is to reduce SSIs. To achieve this goal, the first step is to measure the SSI rates to define the magnitude of the problem. By monitoring SSI rates over time, it is possible to identify potential patient safety problems and promptly implement appropriate interventions. The application of a standardized protocol (e.g., by participating in a surveillance network) allows intra- and interinstitutional comparisons. The purpose of this comparison is to identify and explain the reasons for variations in infection rates.

The timely conveyance of information to relevant stakeholders—surgeons, surgical staffs, other clinicians, infection prevention and control (IPC) professionals, hospital administrators and managers—can alone lead to reductions in the rates of SSIs [2]. Furthermore, the outputs of the surveillance should also be used by institution leaders who can help facilitate change to assure that best and evidence-based practices are in place and that they are appropriately standardized across the facility or health system.

E. Ricchizzi (✉)
Department of Innovation in Healthcare and Social Services, Directorate-General Personal Care, Health and Welfare, Emilia-Romagna Region, Bologna, Italy
e-mail: enrico.ricchizzi@gmail.com

© The Author(s) 2025
S. Bartoli et al. (eds.), *Infections in Surgery*, Updates in Surgery,
https://doi.org/10.1007/978-3-031-60462-1_3

Finally, the SSI surveillance program may include evaluation of the impact of interventions (e.g., antimicrobial prophylaxis protocols or education to reinforce aseptic technique) and monitoring of compliance with recommendations and good practices.

3.1.2   Impact of Surveillance

Several studies demonstrated the positive impact of surveillance in reducing the infection rates. The Study on the Effectiveness of Nosocomial Infection Control found a 32% reduction in healthcare-acquired infections (HAIs) in hospitals with active surveillance programs compared with hospitals without programs [1]. By using standardized definitions, inter- and intrahospital comparison and benchmarking is possible. The effect of interventions can be evaluated over time, allowing identification of potential issues and thus driving cost-effective interventions. Also, it has been proposed that a "surveillance effect" might occur (similar to the Hawthorne effect in clinical trials), that is, "being conscious that one is being observed" may lead to improved practices or adherence to guidelines [3]. Further, the availability of SSI rates could trigger investigations when higher rates compared to baseline are found, leading to the prompt activation of IPC measures. When process indicators are monitored, it is possible to identify the reason for "underperformance" and therefore enact initiatives to improve performance. Participating in an SSI surveillance network allows interhospital comparisons, even though the positive effect on the time trend of SSI rates is controversial given that some studies report a successful reduction in rates after participation [4–6], while others found no effect [7]. It has, however, been observed that the longer the surveillance is in place, the better the SSI rates [8, 9].

3.2   Key Elements of a Surveillance

The surveillance of HAIs is conventionally conducted by passive or active surveillance [10].

Passive surveillance is based on self-reporting of suspected HAIs by the treating physicians. This is a relatively inexpensive strategy since it does not require additional resources to provide adequate information for monitoring trends. However, this is an inefficient method to track HAIs as there is a risk of bias and underreporting, and data quality is difficult to control.

Active surveillance is the systematic collection of data by a designated unbiased surveillance team. The major surveillance networks recommend this method because it provides the most accurate and timely information, although it represents a more resource-consuming approach.

The major SSI surveillance networks worldwide are based on *longitudinal prospective data collection* which requires to follow-up a patient for a period after the surgery. This model allows a wider range of analysis but is resource-consuming. Surveillance can be performed by a *cross-sectional* study in which all the patients are screened for SSI at the same time-point regardless of the time elapsed since the surgical procedure. This model is less resource-demanding but carries a risk of overestimating the infection rates.

3.2.1 Case Definitions

To allow a valid comparison of SSI rates between institutions and over time, standard, valid and reliable definitions must be used. In general, definitions should be meaningful, simple to use, accepted by clinicians, applied consistently and remain stable over time.

Many definitions of SSI are described in literature. However, many authors suggest "there is no single, objective gold standard test for surgical wound infection" [11]. Many published studies are based on Horan et al.'s definitions [12], used in the surveillance of SSIs by the US Centers for Disease Control and Prevention (CDC) [13] and European Centre for Disease Prevention and Control (ECDC) [14].

In these definitions, SSIs are classified as follows:

- *superficial incisional SSIs* involving only skin and subcutaneous tissue of the incision
- *deep incisional SSIs* involving deep soft tissues (fascia and muscles) of the incision
- *organ/space SSIs* involving any part of the body deeper than the fascial/muscle layers that is opened or manipulated during the operative procedure

Definitions may include clinical manifestations (e.g., purulent drainage from the incision, fever), isolation of pathogens from relevant biological specimens, diagnosis by a competent physician (e.g., surgeon). Table 3.1 shows an example of SSI case definitions from the ECDC surveillance system [14].

3.2.2 Methods for Conducting a Surveillance

The gold standard is prospective direct surveillance [15]: healthcare personnel (physician, nurse or IPC professional) observe the surgical site daily starting postoperatively until the end of the follow-up [16]. However, this method is time- and labor-intensive and costly and is often used for research purposes. For routine practice, the indirect method is recommended because it guarantees good accuracy while demanding fewer resources [17]. This method is based on a combination of clinical and administrative data, such as microbiology and medical records, surgeon and/or patient surveys, readmission or re-operation, diagnoses, procedures, operative reports, or antimicrobials prescribed.

Table 3.1 Case definitions of surgical site infections as in the European surveillance system

Superficial incisional	Deep incisional	Organ/space
Infection occurs within 30 days after the operation and involves only skin and subcutaneous tissue of the incision and at least one of the following:	Infection occurs within 30 days after the operation if no implant is left in place or within 90 days if implant is in place and the infection appears to be related to the operation and infection involves deep soft tissue (e.g., fascia, muscle) of the incision and at least one of the following:	Infection occurs within 30 days after the operation if no implant is left in place or within 90 days if implant is in place and the infection appears to be related to the operation and infection involves any part of the anatomy (e.g., organs and spaces) other than the incision that was opened or manipulated during an operation and at least one of the following:
– Purulent drainage with or without laboratory confirmation, from the superficial incision – Organisms isolated from an aseptically obtained culture of fluid or tissue from the superficial incision – At least one of the following signs or symptoms of infection: pain or tenderness, localized swelling, redness, or heat and superficial incision is deliberately opened by surgeon, unless incision is culture-negative – Diagnosis of superficial incisional SSI made by a surgeon or attending physician	– Purulent drainage from the deep incision but not from the organ/space component of the surgical site – A deep incision spontaneously dehisces or is deliberately opened by a surgeon when the patient has at least one of the following signs or symptoms: fever (>38 °C), localized pain or tenderness, unless incision is culture-negative – An abscess or other evidence of infection involving the deep incision is found on direct examination, during reoperation, or by histopathologic or radiologic examination – Diagnosis of deep incisional SSI made by a surgeon or attending physician	– Purulent drainage from a drain that is placed through a stab wound into the organ/space – Organisms isolated from an aseptically obtained culture of fluid or tissue in the organ/space – An abscess or other evidence of infection involving the organ/space that is found on direct examination, during reoperation, or by histopathologic or radiologic examination – Diagnosis of organ/space SSI made by a surgeon or attending physician

SSI surgical site infection
Source: ECDC. Surveillance of surgical site infections and prevention indicators in European hospitals—HAI-Net SSI protocol, version 2.2 [14]

3.2.3   Postdischarge Follow-Up

Despite the known variation among different types of surgery, a significant proportion of SSIs are detected after patient discharge [18]. Most of the superficial incisional SSIs are managed in the outpatient setting; the deep incisional and organ/space infections are typically treated in hospital, in a readmission [19];

implant-associated infections may present until 1 year after the procedure. For these reasons, postdischarge surveillance (PDS) is crucial [20].

There is, however, no known gold standard procedure for PDS [21]. The proportion of SSIs detected through PDS can vary by surveillance method, operative setting, type of SSI, and surgical procedure. Much evidence suggests that an effective strategy should be based on a multifaceted approach [20] since methods based on a single approach, such as the patient questionnaire/interview [22] or surveillance based on ambulatory care settings, have shown insufficient reliability. The use of the combination of electronic medical records, administrative data, and pharmacy dispensing proved to have good predictive values for PDS [23].

To improve comparisons between facilities and minimize potential bias introduced by differences in PDS methods, reporting might be limited to in-hospital non-superficial incisional SSIs relating to the index procedure [15].

The duration of the postoperative follow-up is a fixed period which is defined taking into account the probability of an SSI and the feasibility of the data collection. Major international networks apply a 30-day follow-up, extended to 90 days for prosthetic surgeries.

3.2.4 Surveillance Process

The process starts with the collection of raw data, from which information is extracted, elaborated, and synthesized through an analysis which allows relevant findings to be highlighted for feedback to the stakeholders.

Data collection is the starting point of the process. It is literally the harvest of any useful data sources. Data collection must be structured and follow a written protocol accessible to anyone in the institution. The protocol defines all the items to be collected through definitions that ensure standardization over time and reducing biases from different observers. A prerequisite is to have access to all available information sources. It is essential to focus strictly on information sufficient to meet the surveillance objectives while being sustainable over time. Essential data should include characteristics of the patient, of the surgical procedure and of the SSI. Some surveillance systems also include information about best practices (e.g., antibiotic prophylaxis).

Data management and validation is the second step of the process which is allows building of a complete and reliable database. Missing data, errors and other inconsistencies are cleaned prior to analysis. The data quality indicators help this operation. Periodic validation of the surveillance ensures that the information is consistent with the survey protocol and thus produces reliable results and indicates the need for interventions (e.g., re-training of the surveyors).

Analysis is the phase of extracting information from the data. The routine analysis is based on a plan that answers the objectives of the surveillance. Analysis should include measurement of the magnitude of the events, whilst describing the case-mix of patients and surgical procedures. Both raw and standardized indicators should be provided to allow stronger comparisons and interpretations. Some examples follow.

SSI ratio (or cumulative incidence) is the proportion of surgical procedures in which an SSI was found and is calculated as follows:

$$\text{Percentage of SSIs} = \frac{\text{all first SSIs in that category}}{\text{all operations in that category}} \times 100$$

SSI rate (or incidence density) is the number of SSIs occurring over time and depends on the follow-up. It is calculated as follows:

$$\text{Incidence density of SSIs} = \frac{\text{all first SSIs in that category}}{\text{postoperative patient days with known date end follow-up}} \times 1000$$

The *basic SSI risk index* is used to adjust the risk and assigns surgical patients to categories. It is a composite risk index that captures the joint influence of three major risk factors present at the time of the operation [24, 25]: operation lasting more than the duration cut point; wound contamination class [26]; the patient's ASA classification [27].

Interpretation is the critical reading of results through comparison with reference threshold values, on the knowledge of the organization and personal experience. The purpose of this step is to highlight any critical issues and areas for improvement or to monitor the conditions for patient safety. It must consider any changes in the practice (e.g., improvement actions) or organization that could have an impact on infection rates. A facilitating element is the availability of reference values (benchmarks) such as baseline values and comparison indicators. Information that is not directly available in the surveillance and for which other infrastructures within the organization are responsible should be included. A warm recommendation is to maintain an honest and neutral stance towards the results, avoiding defensive or accusatory attitudes.

3.2.5 Feedback of Results

The outcomes of the surveillance must be communicated to the stakeholders, such as surgeons, staff, and hospital administrators. A surveillance report should include both appropriate rates and counts and a commentary for the results. Data quality indicators (e.g., coverage of the surveillance) and characteristics of the patients and surgical procedures (e.g., risk index) may facilitate correct interpretation. Comparison with reference data (e.g., national benchmark) may help to promote process improvement. Simple reports or dashboards that the target audience can easily understand are very effective. Surveillance reports should be periodically presented to the surgical team to include their comments in the overall interpretation and discuss strategies for preventing infections. During the feedback, suggestions for further requests (e.g., additional analysis) might be presented and could be included in the revision or upgrade of the surveillance.

3.3 Implementation of a Surveillance System

A set of minimal requirements [28] is suggested by the US Association for Professionals in Infection Control and Epidemiology. Among them, a written plan that states goals, objects and elements of the surveillance process is the starting point. The plan must be based on consistent elements of surveillance (e.g., definitions, calculation methods) and include evaluation methods. Furthermore, it is recommended that adequate human resources are allocated to ensure that constant rigor is applied in data collection.

References

1. Haley RW, Quade D, Freeman HE, Bennett JV. The SENIC Project. Study on the efficacy of nosocomial infection control (SENIC Project). Summary of study design. Am J Epidemiol. 1980;111(5):472–85.
2. Gaynes R, Richards C, Edwards J, et al. Feeding back surveillance data to prevent hospital-acquired infections. Emerg Infect Dis. 2001;7(2):295–8.
3. Gastmeier P, Schwab F, Sohr D, et al. Reproducibility of the surveillance effect to decrease nosocomial infection rates. Infect Control Hosp Epidemiol. 2009;30(10):993–9.
4. Astagneau P, L'Hériteau F, Daniel F, et al. Reducing surgical site infection incidence through a network: results from the French ISO-RAISIN surveillance system. J Hosp Infect. 2009;72(2):127–34.
5. Marchi M, Pan A, Gagliotti C, et al. The Italian national surgical site infection surveillance programme and its positive impact, 2009 to 2011. Euro Surveill. 2014;19(21):20815.
6. Brandt C, Sohr D, Behnke M, et al. Reduction of surgical site infection rates associated with active surveillance. Infect Control Hosp Epidemiol. 2006;27(12):1347–51.
7. Staszewicz W, Eisenring MC, Bettschart V, et al. Thirteen years of surgical site infection surveillance in Swiss hospitals. J Hosp Infect. 2014;88(1):40–7.
8. Abbas M, Tartari E, Allegranzi B, et al. The effect of participating in a surgical site infection (SSI) surveillance network on the time trend of SSI rates: a systematic review. Infect Control Hosp Epidemiol. 2017;38(11):1364–6.
9. Vicentini C, Dalmasso P, Politano G, et al. Surgical site infections in Italy, 2009–2015: incidence, trends, and impact of surveillance duration on infection risk. Surg Infect. 2019;20(6):504–9.
10. Sartelli M, Pagani L, Iannazzo S, et al. A proposal for a comprehensive approach to infections across the surgical pathway. World J Emerg Surg. 2020;15(1):13.
11. Bruce J, Russell EM, Mollison J, Krukowski ZH. The quality of measurement of surgical wound infection as the basis for monitoring: a systematic review. J Hosp Infect. 2001;49(2):99–108.
12. Horan TC, Gaynes RP, Martone WJ, et al. CDC definitions of nosocomial surgical site infections, 1992: a modification of CDC definitions of surgical wound infections. Infect Control Hosp Epidemiol. 1992;13(10):606–8.
13. Centers for Disease Control and Prevention—National Healthcare Safety Network. Surgical site infection event. Jan 2023. https://www.cdc.gov/nhsn/pdfs/pscmanual/9pscssicurrent.pdf. Accessed 16 Mar 2024.
14. European Centre for Disease Prevention and Control. Surveillance of surgical site infections and prevention indicators in European hospitals—HAI-Net SSI protocol, version 2.2. Stockholm: ECDC; 2017. https://www.ecdc.europa.eu/sites/default/files/documents/HAI-Net-SSI-protocol-v2.2.pdf. Accessed 16 Mar 2024.
15. Anderson DJ, Podgorny K, Berríos-Torres SI, et al. Strategies to prevent surgical site infections in acute care hospitals: 2014 update. Infect Control Hosp Epidemiol. 2014;35(6):605–27.
16. Condon RE, Schulte WJ, Malangoni MA, et al. Effectiveness of a surgical wound surveillance program. Arch Surg. 1983;118(3):303–7.

17. Cardo DM, Falk PS, Mayhall CG. Validation of surgical wound surveillance. Infect Control Hosp Epidemiol. 1993;14(4):211–5.
18. Holtz TH, Wenzel RP. Postdischarge surveillance for nosocomial wound infection: a brief review and commentary. Am J Infect Control. 1992;20(4):206–13.
19. Ming DY, Chen LF, Miller BA, Anderson DJ. The impact of depth of infection and post-discharge surveillance on rate of surgical-site infections in a network of community hospitals. Infect Control Hosp Epidemiol. 2012;33(3):276–82. Erratum in: Infect Control Hosp Epidemiol. 2013;34(3):333.
20. Manniën J, Wille JC, Snoeren RL, van den Hof S. Impact of postdischarge surveillance on surgical site infection rates for several surgical procedures: results from the nosocomial surveillance network in The Netherlands. Infect Control Hosp Epidemiol. 2006;27(8):809–16.
21. Petherick ES, Dalton JE, Moore PJ, Cullum N. Methods for identifying surgical wound infection after discharge from hospital: a systematic review. BMC Infect Dis. 2006;6:170.
22. Manian FA, Meyer L. Comparison of patient telephone survey with traditional surveillance and monthly physician questionnaires in monitoring surgical wound infections. Infect Control Hosp Epidemiol. 1993;14(4):216–8.
23. Sands K, Vineyard G, Livingston J, et al. Efficient identification of postdischarge surgical site infections: use of automated pharmacy dispensing information, administrative data, and medical record information. J Infect Dis. 1999;179(2):434–41.
24. Haley RW, Culver DH, Morgan WM, et al. Identifying patients at high risk of surgical wound infection. A simple multivariate index of patient susceptibility and wound contamination. Am J Epidemiol. 1985;121(2):206–15.
25. Culver DH, Horan TC, Gaynes RP, et al. Surgical wound infection rates by wound class, operative procedure, and patient risk index. National Nosocomial Infections Surveillance System. Am J Med. 1991;91(3B):152S–7S.
26. Altemeier WABJ, Pruitt BA, Sandusky WR. Manual on control of infection in surgical patients. 2nd ed. Philadelphia, PA: JB Lippincott; 1984.
27. American Society of Anesthesiologists. Statement on ASA physical status classification system (updated 13 Dec 2020). https://www.asahq.org/standards-and-practice-parameters/statement-on-asa-physical-status-classification-system. Accessed 16 Mar 2024.
28. Lee TB, Montgomery OG, Marx J, et al. Recommended practices for surveillance: Association for Professionals in Infection Control and Epidemiology (APIC), Inc. Am J Infect Control. 2007;35(7):427–40.

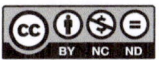

Measuring and Improving Care in Surgical Site Infections

4

Stefano Bartoli, Giulia Ianni, Tommaso Castrucci,
Roberto Gabrielli, Andrea Siani, and Tommaso Bellandi

4.1　Introduction

The probability that a patient is the victim of an adverse event—i.e., suffers damage or discomfort attributable, even if involuntarily, to the medical care provided during the period of hospitalization, which causes an extension of the hospitalization period, failure to recover, a deterioration in health conditions or even death—represents one of the most controversial aspects of medicine and summarizes the commitment for risk managers and healthcare professionals to ensure safety and quality of care, which also necessarily involves all actions useful for preventing or mitigating surgical site infections (SSIs) [1].

Approximately 250 million surgical procedures are performed worldwide every year. While most of these procedures lead to good results and an improvement in patient health, unfortunately not all have such positive outcomes. Healthcare-associated infections (HAIs) have a significant clinical and economic impact: they are responsible for extending the length of hospitalization (about 16 million additional hospital days at European level), increasing the resistance of microorganisms to antibiotics and causing significant mortality and long-term disability, with a major direct and indirect economic impact on both the system and the patients and their families, amounting to over 7 billion euros in Europe. The prevalence of HAIs in acute care hospitals is 8%, with high variability between hospital departments (from 22.9% in intensive care to 1.3% in psychiatry) [2, 3].

S. Bartoli (✉) · G. Ianni · T. Castrucci · R. Gabrielli · A. Siani
Department of Vascular Surgery, Sant'Eugenio Hospital-ASL Roma 2, Rome, Italy
e-mail: steba08@gmail.com; giuliaianni@hotmail.com; tcastrucci@gmail.com; roberto.gabrielli@aslroma2.it; andreasiani@yahoo.it

T. Bellandi
Patient Safety Unit, AUSL Toscana Nordovest-Cittadella della Salute, Lucca, Italy
e-mail: tommasobellandi@gmail.com

© The Author(s) 2025
S. Bartoli et al. (eds.), *Infections in Surgery*, Updates in Surgery,
https://doi.org/10.1007/978-3-031-60462-1_4

SSI is one of the most undesirable and potentially very serious outcomes of surgery and represents one of the five negative events that characterize HAIs. The World Health Organization (WHO) data report that SSIs are a significant part of the global public health problem of HAIs [4].

The idea of preventing HAIs is reflected in the well-known admonition to doctors to "First, do no harm", which is a cornerstone of the Hippocratic Oath. Infections that occur in association with hospital care are therapeutically, organizationally, and economically demanding. They reflect an organizational deviation from good practices that invite us to adequately evaluate some intrinsic characteristics of the patient or of the environment in which he is hospitalized, such as comorbidities like diabetes and obesity, or performing a nasal swab to decolonize the nose or a preoperative shower with antibacterial soap—simple but proven effective measures.

According to some studies, 50% of HAIs could be prevented through the adoption of adequate surveillance systems and prevention programs. Hand hygiene is the most cost-effective antimicrobial stewardship intervention, which allows us to save many human lives and economic resources calculated in about 1000 days of hospitalization avoided per year per 100,000 people [5].

4.2   Barriers to Surgical Site Infections Prevention

While significant progress has been made in infection prevention and control, one of the limiting factors in SSI prevention is the often subjective and uneven implementation of recommended prevention practices due to low awareness of the problem, which is viewed more as episodic and not related to systemic factors.

In fact, practices of proven efficacy are often not adopted and, when they are, their adoption is discontinuous or inhomogeneous due to a lack of leadership and resources and often the inability of surgical teams to commit to providing safer care.

The widespread adoption of the WHO SSI prevention guidelines will certainly increase surgical safety: the implementation of checklists for monitoring what we have decided to keep under control to reduce surgery-related infections, to be applied to the patient population in all perioperative phases and which outline exactly what to do pre-, intra-, and postoperatively to prevent SSI. It is not necessary to apply all the recommendations but, by analyzing one's own situation, one can define the criticalities and on those apply the relative recommendations by implementing a monitoring system [6, 7].

Achieving a culture of safety requires an understanding of the values, attitudes, beliefs, and norms that are important to healthcare organizations and the appropriate and expected attitudes and behaviors for patient safety. As reported by Øvretveit [8], few studies have evaluated the effect of context on the implementation of safety and quality interventions in the health sector defined by the literature for some time now among sectors with high complexity and risk due to multidisciplinarity and multi-professionalism, process variability, high degree of innovation, high frequency of emergencies and uncertainty of medical practice, as well as patient vulnerability, with a spectrum of complexity ranging from attention to the labeling of similar drugs or with confusing names (LASA: "Look-Alike/Sound-Alike") to the need to integrate multidisciplinary skills for the management of more complex cases [9].

In the analysis, consider the prevalence of errors and the possibility of avoiding them, as well as the different detection strategies. For example, between what follows from a sepsis compared to the ability to intercept the presence of antibiotic-resistant germs in frail patients, especially if elderly and with multiple hospitalizations or coming from other healthcare facilities.

There are many barriers to implementing simple actions to prevent or mitigate the risk of SSI, the most frequently reported being: inadequately redistributed workloads, lack of time or human resources, poor communication, inadequate organizational skills, insufficient leadership effectiveness, inadequate efforts to keep up with standards, underestimation of teamwork.

Certainly, the continuing professional fragmentation and the lack of teamwork goals, by leaving the different care specialists to continue to work in a "silos manner", further contribute to the risk of errors in the health care system, as noted by Hignett et al. [10] in their study of the system's barriers to effective health care delivery. Poor or disrupted communication (due respectively to a fragmented work structure and a poorly designed physical environment) presents additional barriers to effective and safe practice [11].

There is still a need to develop effective and appropriate reporting and learning systems which, when introduced in conjunction with the right culture, can play an important role in identifying systemic weaknesses, which Woods and Cook [12] advocate as the most effective recovery from errors, compared to the identification of problematic or "defective" people.

Lack of feedback and improvement actions following an incident report is recognized as the most relevant barrier in an Italian survey of healthcare workers [13].

Blaming people for errors usually caused by flawed systems creates anxiety and fear in the staff and can change the way people work. A fair and just culture is one in which leaders and staff members learn and improve by openly identifying and examining their weaknesses and opportunities for improvement [14].

4.3   Systems Engineering Initiative for Patient Safety

The promotion of patient safety requires a systematic approach and the adoption of diversified methods and tools, in relation to the specific purposes, the sociocultural and organizational context, and progress of the culture of safety. Only in this way can clinical risk analysis become a driver of sustainability by shifting attention from cost dynamics to investment dynamics, thus promoting the value of actions to reduce the risk of SSI.

To these considerations, we need to add another theoretical and methodological assumption which, although technically and scientifically consolidated, has not yet been fully applied in the context of risk management in health services. This further assumption concerns the definition of the systemic approach, for which it is necessary to have a clear, valid, and reliable reference model that is sensitive to the peculiarities of the contexts in which healthcare is provided. The Systems Engineering Initiative for Patient Safety (SEIPS) model responds to this need, as it has been developed and applied for almost three decades in many areas of healthcare services at an international level [15].

The model has its roots in the science of human factors and ergonomics (HFE) and is based on the study and improvement of interactions between the human, technological and organizational components of a work system, through the combination of techniques and tools of quantitative and qualitative analysis of human activities. The goal is to design and create work and living environments, as well as person-centered technological and organizational tools aimed at improving the system's performance, while respecting the health and safety of individuals and communities. In the context of industry and services, including the healthcare sector, the analysis of the system always starts from real contexts, from work as it is, in comparison with more formal approaches that start from the analysis of work as it is imagined in official documents.

Both the analysis and the ergonomic interventions of research and practice can be applied at several levels of the system [16, 17]:

- *macro level*—political, social and regulatory context, resource availability and constraints
- *meso level*—organization and management of the production system
- *micro level*—conducting activities, making decisions, taking action and verifying real contexts

SEIPS offers a relatively simple reference scheme for both analysis and planning, as it expands and details the classic functional model of organizations described through the structure-process-results triad, emphasizing the decisive role of interactions between the components of the structure in determining processes and outcomes, as well as the retroactive effects that these have on the same structure of interactions. This reading of the dual dynamics of the system is the added value of SEIPS compared to other models, which is well suited to describe the genesis of problems that impact on patient safety, both positively and negatively.

Applied to safety in surgery and in particular to the prevention of infections within a healthcare organization, a surgical department or a single surgical operating unit, SEIPS allows us to explore: the critical interactions between people, the tasks they perform, the rules that govern them, the tools used and the work environment; the good practices that facilitate the performance of the activities and the achievement of favorable outcomes for the patient (e.g., treatment of the disease, safety in the results, quality of the experience), for the clinicians (e.g., clinical effectiveness, reputation, learning) and for the organization (e.g., appropriateness, efficiency, image); the bad practices that hinder the achievement of results and undermine the quality of processes and patients' and workers' safety.

4.4 Planning and Implementing a Surveillance Program

Surveillance of surgical care and SSI is a critical component of an infection prevention and control program. By helping to identify risk factors for SSI, surveillance contributes to drive behavior change actions throughout the system with a multidisciplinary and multiprofessional approach.

Surgical procedures vary in their risk of infection, and procedures can be included in the surveillance plan based on a list of criteria, such as: potential consequences of infections, cost of treatment, particular clinical concern of surgeons, specific demands of the infection prevention team. The surveillance plan will therefore focus on procedures identified during the risk assessment by analyzing those procedures that are high volume, high risk or subject to problems or those that are of particular interest to the organization, defining the objectives of the monitoring accordingly and collecting data accordingly.

A critical step in developing a surveillance program for SSI is the selection of procedures to be monitored. Thus, in addition to measuring infection rates, attention to rates of compliance with established infection prevention policies (e.g., maintenance of normothermia, fluid volumes, and appropriate technique for applying skin antiseptics) will be important.

Surgical patient care involves multiple processes designed to prevent surgical infections. In the preoperative phase, hand hygiene, careful assessment of the patient's status and risk factors, and the initiation of specific procedures, such as maintaining normothermia, are examples of these infection prevention processes. Intraoperatively, infection prevention processes include skin antisepsis with proven detergent disinfectants, maintenance of normothermia, and glucose monitoring. Postoperatively, aseptic wound care is a primary prevention process [18].

Patients identified as "at risk" will then receive measures to prevent SSI according to the organization's best practice protocol. For example, protocols could be set up for reviewing nutrition, checking detergent disinfectants used preoperatively, monitoring intraoperative and postoperative blood glucose, or maintaining normothermia. The important thing is that each of these steps in the process can be monitored and measured. Over time, as an appropriate sample size is developed, one can begin to identify which steps in the process are the most critical to preventing negative outcomes. Paul Batalden argued that: "Every system is perfectly designed to get the results it gets": if one does not have a well-designed process for preventing SSI, it should not be surprising that there is no process for change [19].

By tracking the process measurements, the root cause of the system failure can be found. For example, one may find that there is a shortage of methicillin nasal ointments that reduce nasal colonization by *Staphylococcus aureus* and infections, or that a risk assessment has not been done for every patient that is admitted, or that operating room temperature controls are not constantly monitored. Whatever the problem, however, it can be identified, evaluated, and possibly fixed.

Providing information on surgeon-specific SSI rates can raise awareness among surgeons by encouraging them to better analyze their patients' conditions, but also to define different attitudes towards colleagues working in the same department and performing similar surgical procedures.

During surveillance to identify and classify SSI, we collect data from various sources, including: the medical record with all its descriptive parts (clinical and nursing diary), laboratory cultures and blood chemistry tests with the specific infection markers, as well as radiology and pathology reports. Then we have all the information from patients and caregivers, reports of conditions predisposing to an SSI. It is then necessary to inspect the wound during the follow-up and record its condition, aware that most SSIs, according to the NHS Institute for Innovation and Improvement criteria, occur within 30–90 days of the surgical procedure and are still considered as associated with the treatment [20].

Once acquired the data, it is necessary to identify and analyze the clinical cases and risk situations that deserve further study, to establish possible actions for local or system improvement. Below, we present an integrated path of reporting analysis and prevention of significant events for patient safety, which integrate the classic methods of infection prevention and control with those developed in the field of risk management.

4.5   Reporting and Learning from Significant Events

To successfully assess risks, a reporting and learning system should be in place to allow the recognition of actual and potential issues. Staff should feel free to report these risk issues without repercussion. For example, if observing and monitoring surgical scrubbing reveals incomplete or unsystematic execution by the operating table personnel, then members of the observation team should feel free to report this behavior, so as to be able to implement corrective measures (timer, adequate scrubbing instruments, retraining on the importance of surgical scrubbing, etc.). Or, if the instruments arriving in the operating room do not comply with the standards defined in the procedure (altered or inadequately stored kit, etc.), the system must allow for anomalies to be reported immediately so as to make corrections and/or consider reprogramming of the sterilization cycles.

Reported risk cases or situations should be reviewed and analyzed on an ongoing basis, trends identified, and significant individual events noted and followed up by audits involving staff highlighting what has been reported and the specific actions deemed necessary. Evidence should be shared with relevant staff and coordinators, as aggregated data without identifiers, and staff and leadership should work together to remedy potential risks [21].

Some serious events are defined as "sentinel events". According to the Joint Commission, a sentinel event is an unexpected event resulting in death or serious physical or psychological injury, or risk thereof, thus including any process variation for which a recurrence would carry a significant probability of a serious adverse outcome. Such events are called sentinel events, signaling the need for immediate investigation and response. For example, in surgical services a sentinel event might be unexpected death in the operating room from septic shock.

Requirements related to the management of sentinel events usually include root cause analysis or systems analysis to determine the timeline of the facts leading to the adverse outcome, evaluate active failures and contributory risk factors and establish an action plan to reduce the probability of event recurrence. This type of analysis is effective when it is focused on systems and not individuals. A systems analysis includes examining the interactions between human factors, equipment, environmental factors, human resources, information management, and leadership and communication issues. The goal is to get to the more relevant contributory factors of the incident so as to identify where improvement can make a difference.

The Safety Walk Round (SWR) is another risk assessment technique, which integrates field visits with hospital managers and structured interviews with healthcare personnel on critical issues and best practices for patient safety. SWR engages managers in open patient safety discussions with frontline workers to foster an open communication-based safety culture, motivating and involving leaders and staff in actions for patient safety and it monitors the actual correct implementation of clinical risk management procedures and indicators [22].

The interviews, with individuals or groups, are aimed at identifying the current or potential risks that can lead to adverse events for patients and the measures that, according to the various stakeholders, could be usefully introduced to prevent their occurrence and guarantee the safety of the patient. The SWR therefore allows the assessment of system vulnerabilities and the adoption, even in a short time, of preventive measures, while promoting the mutual commitment of operators and managers to implementing improvements for the development of a culture of safety.

The SWR is widely used and has proven effective in developing a culture of safety, as well as contributing to the proactive identification of risks and adverse events and the adoption of improvement strategies at all levels of the organization. Although in our country the application of this method is still in its infancy, it should be considered that it can count on the habit of some managers of "walking around" the hospital units to learn about the problems personally.

It is therefore a question of planning its use: organizing visits in a structured and systematic way, applying a rigorous methodology, which includes preparation, the actual walk-round of the unit, collection and processing of available data, analysis and definition of priorities, identification of improvement strategies, their implementation and subsequent assessment.

In the facilities in which SWR are regularly carried out, the professionals' commitment to safety increases, thanks to an improvement in the organizational climate, which facilitates the commitment to quality development and the search for a consensus in the choice of areas for improvement [23].

The method should be carried out as a peer review and the results reported to a peer committee. The transition from promoting a culture of safety to monitoring the ability to be resilient so as to create focus on certain priorities/areas of application, involve management in the preparation and feedback, and where possible use an external point of view and skills, and involve patient representatives [24].

Finally, a quality improvement model allows an organization to define, structure and implement improvements in a coherent way. This consistency promotes staff understanding and clarifies roles. A performance improvement model that is used repeatedly and that is familiar to all surgical services makes improvements easier to conduct, and each organization should select the model that best works for it.

4.6   Conclusion

Many of the current limitations to the creation of a culture of patient safety in the operating room derive from a lack of leadership, both at management levels, due to a lack of structured and lasting plans, and locally, due to a lack of awareness of the problems and low confidence in change. Strong and transparent leadership is essential to ensure effective acceptance of safety activities by all members of the healthcare team and to implement and incorporate these practices into the daily work routine.

Healthcare systems, including the Italian one, are moving at greater speed in the fight against HAI and antibiotic resistance: it is time to harmonize standards at regional and hospital level with guidelines defined at national level and to use evidence-based protocols and specific indicators at the local level, strengthening the monitoring and performance appraisal tools.

For this reason, it is necessary to strengthen and integrate health information systems at local and regional level, with attention to the bidirectionality of information flows (collection and return of data to interested parties) so as to increase the levels of awareness and of information/education for health professionals, citizens and all players in the health system.

Measuring performance through generalized outcomes, such as in-hospital mortality, infection rates, and medication errors is common practice. Such measures represent key values in institutional sustainability and care delivery practice, but do not capture all dimensions that matter most to the patient [25]. Value-based initiatives are increasingly gaining prominence as strategic models of healthcare management, which requires an in-depth exploration of how to integrate the patient experience of professionals into SSI prevention and risk management as well [26].

What happened in the dramatic years of the Covid-19 pandemic has also made it a priority to work towards integrating infection prevention and control activities in healthcare facilities and communities, with healthcare risk management activities, with a particular attention to frail patients [26]. Both activities, divided into distinct functions within healthcare organizations, which have emerged over time and relate to different cultures of reference, are aimed at patient safety and can certainly contribute to improving the organization and management of healthcare services if they recognize and share their respective competencies in a common framework.

On the one hand, patient safety can contribute to:

- increase awareness of risk factors and possible improvement actions through the reporting and accurate analysis of infections that are related to healthcare and are therefore subject to reporting and analysis with audits of significant events, or mortality and morbidity reviews.

- strengthen the application of prevention and protection measures for patients and operators by sharing and developing bundles of good practices for the prevention of infections, including those of surgical wounds, according to the cooperative logic of the community of practices.

On the other hand, infection prevention and control can further develop:

- formative peer assessment of infection prevention practices and evaluation control according to clear and measurable standards by management.
- clinical surveillance and advanced epidemiological investigations with the support of state-of-the-art information technology systems that make it possible to promptly alert healthcare professionals and management in the presence of a case of HAI or an emerging germ and to analyze trends at a territorial or organizational level.

All this, with a strong involvement of individual patients and communities in the application of good practices as well as widespread surveillance, which requires commitments at all levels for education and training. For example, for the prevention of surgical wound infections, the careful adherence of the patient and his family to the healthcare team's recommendations at the time of discharge is of fundamental importance to avoid contamination and treat the wound effectively.

It is a perspective that can find integration in a corporate risk management system, supported in Italy by law 24/2017 which commits healthcare organizations and professionals to identify, analyze and prevent all health risks [26], therefore including those associated with HAIs, as well as at European and international level by plans to combat infections associated with multi-resistant microorganisms.

References

1. Kohn LT, Corrigan JM, Donaldson MS, editors. To err is human. Building a safer health system. Washington, DC: National Academies Press; 1999.
2. Mehtar S, Wanyoro A, Ogunsola F, et al. Implementation of surgical site infection surveillance in low- and middle-income countries: a position statement for the International Society for Infectious Diseases. Int J Infect Dis. 2020;100:123–31.
3. Seidelman JL, Mantyh CR, Anderson DJ. Surgical site infection prevention: a review. JAMA. 2023;329(3):244–52.
4. European Centre for Disease Prevention and Control. Healthcare-associated infections: surgical site infections. In: ECDC. Annual epidemiological report for 2018–2020. Stockholm: ECDC; 2023. https://www.ecdc.europa.eu/en/publications-data/healthcare-associated-infections-surgical-site-annual-2018-2020. Accessed 16 Mar 2024.
5. World Health Organization—Organisation for Economic Co-operation and Development. Addressing the burden of infections and antimicrobial resistance associated with healthcare—focus on G7 countries. WHO–OECD; 2022. https://www.oecd.org/els/health-systems/Antimicrobial-Resistance-in-G7-Countries-and-Beyond.pdf. Accessed 16 Mar 2024.
6. Skoufalos A, Clarke JL, Napp M, et al. Improving awareness of best practices to reduce surgical site infection: a multistakeholder approach. Am J Med Qual. 2012;27(4):297–304.

7. World Health Organization. Preventing surgical site infections: implementation approaches for evidence-based recommendations. Geneva: WHO; 2018. https://www.who.int/publications/i/item/9789241514385. Accessed 16 Mar 2024.
8. Øvretveit J. Understanding the conditions for improvement: research to discover which context influences affect improvement success. BMJ Qual Saf. 2011;20(Suppl_1):i18–23.
9. World Health Organization. Advanced infection prevention and control training—prevention of surgical site infection: trainer's guide. 2018. https://cdn.who.int/media/docs/default-source/integrated-health-services-(ihs)/ssi/training/ssi-trainers-guide.pdf. Accessed 16 Mar 2024.
10. Hignett S, Lang A, Pickup L, et al. More holes than cheese. What prevents the delivery of effective, high quality and safe health care in England? Ergonomics. 2018;61(1):5–14.
11. Donaldson L, Ricciardi W, Sheridan S, Tartaglia R, editors. Textbook of patient safety and clinical risk management. Springer Nature; 2020.
12. Woods D, Cook R. Nine steps to move forward from error. Cogn Tech Work. 2002;4:137–44.
13. Albolino S, Tartaglia R, Bellandi T, et al. Patient safety and incident reporting: survey of Italian healthcare workers. Qual Saf Health Care. 2010;19(Suppl 3):i8–i12.
14. Dagliana G, Albolino S, Mulissa Z, et al. From theory to real-world integration: implementation science and beyond. In: Donaldson L, Ricciardi W, Sheridan S, Tartaglia R, editors. Textbook of patient safety and clinical risk management. Springer Nature; 2020.
15. Carayon P, Schoofs Hundt A, Karsh BT, et al. Work system design for patient safety: the SEIPS model. Qual Saf Health Care. 2006;15(Suppl 1):i50–8.
16. Carayon P, Bass E, Bellandi T, et al. Socio-technical systems analysis in health care: a research agenda. IIE Trans Healthc Syst Eng. 2011;1(1):145–60.
17. Bellandi T, Albolino S. Human factors and ergonomics for a safe transition to digital health. Stud Health Technol Inform. 2019;265:12–21.
18. Soule BM. Evidence-based principles and practices for preventing surgical site infection. Joint Commission International; 2018. https://store.jointcommissioninternational.org/assets/3/7/JCI_SSI_Toolkit.pdf. Accessed 16 Mar 2024.
19. McInnis D. What system? Dartmouth Med. 2006;30(4). https://dartmed.dartmouth.edu/summer06/html/what_system.php. Accessed 16 Mar 2024.
20. Clarke J, Davidge M, James L. The how-to guide for measurement for improvement. NHS Institute for Innovation and Improvement; 2010. https://www.england.nhs.uk/improvement-hub/wp-content/uploads/sites/44/2017/11/How-to-Guide-for-Measurement-for-Improvement.pdf. Accessed 16 Mar 2024.
21. Tocco Tussardi I, Moretti F, Capasso M, et al. Improving the culture of safety among healthcare workers: integration of different instruments to gain major insights and drive effective changes. Int J Health Plann Manag. 2022;37(1):429–51.
22. Poletti P. Safety walkaround. Care. 2009;11(2):27–33. https://careonline.it/wp-content/uploads/2008/08/care_2_09.pdf. Accessed 16 Mar 2024.
23. Machen S. Thematic reviews of patient safety incidents as a tool for systems thinking: a quality improvement report. BMJ Open Qual. 2023;12(2):e002020.
24. Zanotto BS, Beck da Silva Etges AP, Zago Marcolino MA, Polanczyk CA. Value-based healthcare initiatives in practice: a systematic review. J Healthc Manag. 2021;66(5):340–65.
25. World Health Organization. Implications of the COVID-19 pandemic for patient safety: a rapid review. Geneva: WHO; 2022. https://iris.who.int/bitstream/handle/10665/361283/9789240055094-eng.pdf. Accessed 16 Mar 2024.
26. Bellandi T, Tartaglia R, Sheikh A, Donaldson L. Italy recognises patient safety as a fundamental right. BMJ. 2017;357:j2277.

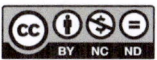

Principles of Infection Prevention and Control in Surgery

5

Antonella Agodi

5.1 Introduction

Surgical site infections (SSIs) are potential complications that can arise from any surgical procedure. Preventing these infections is a complex task that requires the integration of multiple measures before, during, and after surgery. In general, infection prevention and control (IPC) is a practical and evidence-based approach aimed at protecting patients and healthcare workers from preventable infections. It requires consistent action at all levels of the healthcare system, involving policymakers, healthcare workers, and individuals seeking healthcare services. IPC holds unique significance in patient safety and quality of care, as it is universally applicable to every healthcare interaction, encompassing both providers and recipients of care. Failure in implementing effective IPC measures can lead to harm and even fatalities. Thus, achieving high-quality healthcare delivery is impossible without robust IPC practices [1]. Existing guidelines provide recommendations and best practices for healthcare professionals to reduce the risk of SSIs [2–6]. In 2016, the World Health Organization (WHO) also published its *Global Guidelines for the Prevention of Surgical Site Infection*, which provide recommendations applicable to various healthcare settings worldwide. These WHO guidelines, which were updated in 2018, aim to standardize preoperative, intraoperative, and postoperative measures and provide evidence-based recommendations to prevent SSIs [7].

A. Agodi (✉)

Department of Medical and Surgical Sciences and Advanced Technologies G.F. Ingrassia, University of Catania, Catania, Italy
e-mail: agodia@unict.it

S. Bartoli et al. (eds.), *Infections in Surgery*, Updates in Surgery,
https://doi.org/10.1007/978-3-031-60462-1_5

5.2 Surveillance

Surveillance of healthcare-associated infections (HAIs) is a critical component of an effective IPC program [8–10]. As defined by the WHO, surveillance is the continuous and systematic collection, analysis, interpretation, and evaluation of health data. It is closely integrated with the timely dissemination of these data to those who need it for informed decision-making [11]. When it comes to defining SSI, there is a lack of consensus, and numerous definitions have been proposed. A systematic review revealed a substantial number of definitions, with more than one-third of the included studies adopting the definition provided by the Centers for Disease Control and Prevention (CDC) [4]. In addition, many countries employ the HAI SSI protocol developed by the European Centre for Disease Prevention and Control (ECDC) [12]. These standardized protocols enable consistent monitoring and comparison of SSI rates across different healthcare settings [4, 12].

The primary objective of surveillance is to collect data on SSIs to assess the extent of the problem. These data are then analyzed to identify trends and patterns, enabling a thorough interpretation of the findings. Surveillance data play a crucial role in guiding the identification of improvement strategies and evaluating the effectiveness of implemented interventions. Providing feedback on SSI rates to relevant stakeholders holds significant importance [8]. The surveillance of SSI is a fundamental component of the WHO safe surgery guidelines [13]. To facilitate inter-hospital comparisons and benchmarking, national networks and collaborative networks, such as the CDC's National Healthcare Safety Network (NHSN), the ECDC's Healthcare-Associated Infections Surveillance Network (HAI-Net), and the International Nosocomial Infection Control Consortium, have been established [14–16].

Successful surveillance programs can contribute to reducing SSI rates in multiple ways. Firstly, the feedback provided to healthcare institutions can prompt investigations into the underlying causes of higher infection rates. It is also worth considering that a "surveillance effect" may occur, where the mere knowledge of being observed can independently lead to improved practices and adherence to guidelines [17]. In addition to the standard practice of prospective surveillance, there is growing evidence that repeated prevalence surveys offer a feasible and efficient approach to assess the burden of SSIs. These surveys can be conducted on a larger scale, at a faster pace, and at a lower cost, making them a valuable method for evaluating the prevalence of SSIs [18, 19]. A substantial proportion of SSIs are believed to be detected after patients have been discharged. Infections associated with implants may not manifest until up to a year after the procedure. Consequently, many surveillance networks recommend the implementation of postdischarge surveillance [20].

5.3 Environment in the Operating Room and Decontamination of Medical Devices

Recent evidence has highlighted the significance of a contaminated healthcare environment in the spread of infections [21]. The operating room (OR) requires thorough daily cleaning, which should be performed before any disinfection process to remove dirt and debris, enhancing the effectiveness of chemical disinfectants. A neutral detergent solution is recommended for effective cleaning, preventing the formation of biofilms, and maximizing disinfectant efficacy.

Proper mechanical ventilation is essential to prevent contamination of surgical wounds from unfiltered air and to remove microorganisms shed in skin scales [22]. While some guidelines have provided recommendations concerning OR ventilation systems [23], several others do not specifically address this topic. The guidance ranges from technical advice on proper air management in the OR [24] to leaving the issue unresolved [25]. Given the low-quality evidence available on the effects of laminar airflow in reducing SSI rates, the WHO Guidelines Development Group suggests that laminar airflow ventilation systems should not be utilized for the purpose of reducing the risk of SSIs in patients undergoing total arthroplasty surgery, emphasizing the need for further research [7]. It is important to consider other factors that could counteract the potential benefits of the ventilation system, such as the frequency of door openings and the presence of individuals inside the OR during surgical procedures [26].

Decontamination of reusable medical devices and patient care equipment is a specialized process governed by established guidelines and standards at national and international levels. The WHO/Pan American Health Organization (PAHO) has produced a manual to guide decontamination and reprocessing activities in healthcare facilities, supporting efforts to improve standards of care [27]. The increasing use of endoscopes requires effective decontamination to protect patients, ensure diagnostic quality, and prolong equipment life [28]. Proper cleaning, disinfection, or sterilization methods should be followed, considering the manufacturer's instructions and compatibility of the decontamination process with the endoscope.

5.4   Preoperative Measures

Preoperative measures for the prevention of SSIs include, but are not limited to preoperative bathing, hair removal, screening and decolonization of *Staphylococcus aureus*, optimal timing for preoperative surgical antibiotic prophylaxis (SAP), and skin preparation [7].

Preoperative whole-body bathing is widely recommended as a beneficial clinical practice to achieve optimal skin cleanliness before surgery, with the aim of reducing bacterial presence, particularly at the incision site. Typically, an antimicrobial soap, such as one containing 4% chlorhexidine gluconate (CHG) combined with a detergent or a triclosan preparation, is utilized for this purpose [29]. Hair removal from the intended surgical incision site has long been a routine step in the preoperative preparation of patients scheduled for surgery. Hair removal should be performed using clippers instead of shaving to minimize the risk of creating small wounds that could harbor bacteria [30].

Staphylococcal infections are common in hospitalized patients and can lead to serious complications, such as postoperative wound infections, hospital-acquired pneumonia, and catheter-related bloodstream infections [31]. Nasal carriage of *S. aureus* has emerged as a well-established risk factor for subsequent infection in various patient populations [32]. The recommended decolonization process involves the administration of mupirocin ointment with mupirocin ointment with or without CHG body wash [33].

The use of antibiotic prophylaxis is recommended in all SSI prevention guidelines provided by professional societies and national authorities [2, 3, 23, 34]. The goal of SAP is to administer the antimicrobial agent at effective concentrations to the surgical site prior to contamination. However, existing recommendations on SAP [6, 23, 35, 36] are not based on systematic reviews, meta-analyses, or rigorous evaluations of the available evidence regarding SAP effectiveness. The WHO Guidelines Development Group performed a comprehensive systematic review, which found no definitive evidence of either benefit or harm when comparing antibiotic administration within 60 min or between 60 and 120 min before the surgical incision. Thus, in the absence of robust evidence, the WHO guidelines recommend the administration of SAP within 120 min before incision, while considering the half-life of the antibiotic [7]. A systematic review of RCTs has indicated that administering additional doses of antibiotics does not effectively reduce the risk of infection [37]. As a result, guidelines suggest discontinuing antibiotic prophylaxis once the surgical wound is closed [7]. A systematic review commissioned by the ECDC has identified five crucial SAP modalities, along with process indicators to monitor their implementation. These modalities encompass the following: establishing a multidisciplinary team to develop, implement, and update a SAP protocol; conducting compliance audits and providing feedback; ensuring administration of SAP within 60 min prior to incision; assigning responsibility for timely administration to the anesthesiologist; administering a single dose of SAP only; and discontinuing SAP at the conclusion of surgery [38].

Before the first operation, the team should thoroughly wash their hands, using a single-use brush or pick for the nails, followed by the application of an antiseptic solution or an alcoholic hand rub. This helps maintain a clean and sterile environment in the OR [39]. Surgical site preparation involves treating the patient's intact skin in the OR before the surgical incision. Commonly used agents for this purpose are chlorhexidine gluconate (CHG) and povidone-iodine (PVP-I) in alcohol-based solutions. Several guidelines recommend the use of alcohol-based solutions for surgical site preparation [5, 23, 36]. The WHO Guidelines Development Group performed a comprehensive systematic review, which found that the use of alcohol-based CHG is beneficial in reducing SSI rates compared to alcohol-based PVP-I [7].

5.5   Perioperative and/or Intraoperative Measures

Ensuring optimal body temperature, oxygenation, glycemic level, hydration, tissue perfusion, and nutritional status are vital components throughout the entire perioperative period.

Hypothermia, characterized by a core temperature below 36 °C, often occurs during and after extensive surgical procedures lasting over 2 h. Accordingly, the WHO recommends the implementation of warming devices in the OR and during the surgical procedure to ensure adequate patient body warming. This aligns with previous healthcare bundles and guidelines aimed at maintaining patient temperature within a safe range [23, 36, 40–44].

Perioperative oxygenation is also emphasized in clinical practice guidelines provided by professional societies and national authorities [5, 23, 42–44]. According to WHO recommendations, adult patients undergoing general anesthesia with tracheal intubation for surgical procedures should receive an 80% fraction of inspired oxygen (FiO_2) intraoperatively. Additionally, if feasible, maintaining this level of oxygenation in the immediate postoperative period for 2–6 h is recommended to minimize the risk of SSIs [7].

Optimal wound healing and resistance to infection rely on adequate tissue oxygenation, which can be enhanced by maintaining appropriate arterial oxygen levels. The WHO Guidelines Development Group has recommended the implementation of goal-directed fluid therapy (GDFT) during surgery as a means to reduce the risk of SSI. GDFT involves individualized fluid administration based on specific patient parameters and goals, aiming to optimize tissue perfusion and oxygenation [7].

During and after surgery, blood glucose levels tend to increase due to the physiological stress caused by the procedure. Several organizations have provided recommendations regarding the control of blood glucose levels during the perioperative period. To reduce the risk of SSIs, the WHO recommendations suggest implementing protocols for intensive perioperative blood glucose control for both diabetic and non-diabetic adult patients undergoing surgical procedures [7].

Several studies have demonstrated the potential benefits of early nutritional support in improving outcomes and reducing infectious complications in specific groups of malnourished or severely injured patients undergoing major surgery [45, 46]. Among the existing guidelines, the WHO stands out as the only one suggesting the consideration of oral or enteral administration of multiple nutrient-enhanced nutritional formulas for underweight patients undergoing major surgical procedures as a means to prevent SSIs [7].

When it comes to the use of immunosuppressive agents, which are frequently prescribed to prevent organ rejection in transplant patients or to treat inflammatory diseases, there is a scarcity of comprehensive and consistent recommendations. The WHO guidelines recommend against the discontinuation of immunosuppressive medication prior to surgery for the specific purpose of preventing SSIs [7]. The decision to discontinue immunosuppressive medication should be made on an individual basis, taking into account the patient's overall condition and the specific risks and benefits associated with their particular situation [7].

The intraoperative period and the moment of incision are equally crucial for reducing the risk of SSIs. The WHO guidelines provide recommendations for this stage, emphasizing the use of sterile, disposable non-woven or sterile reusable woven drapes and gowns. Additionally, these guidelines suggest employing wound protector devices during abdominal surgeries categorized as clean-contaminated, contaminated, or dirty. In contrast, there are no specific recommendations regarding the use of surgical gloves, such as double gloving, changing gloves during the operation, or using a particular type of glove. Similarly, there are no guidelines regarding the practice of changing surgical instruments to a new set of sterile instruments at the time of closure [7].

Intraoperative wound irrigation is a commonly practiced technique among surgeons to prevent SSIs. It involves the application of a solution to the open wound surface to promote wound hydration [47]. The WHO Guidelines Development Group has determined that there is insufficient evidence to support or discourage the use of saline irrigation for incisional wounds before closure to prevent SSIs. However, the panel suggests considering the use of an aqueous PVP-I solution for wound irrigation prior to closure, particularly in clean and clean-contaminated wounds. On the other hand, the panel advises against the use of antibiotic incisional wound irrigation before closure for the purpose of preventing SSIs [7].

Negative Pressure Wound Therapy (NPWT) involves the use of a sealed system connected to a vacuum pump, which applies negative pressure to the wound surface [48–50]. Considering the available evidence, the WHO guidelines suggest the utilization of prophylactic NPWT in adult patients with primarily closed surgical incisions, particularly in high-risk wounds [7].

Surgical suture material is utilized to effectively bring together the wound edges, placing it in direct contact with the wound itself. To prevent microbial colonization of the sutures in surgical incisions, the WHO recommendation is to use triclosan-coated sutures as a measure to reduce the risk of SSIs, regardless of the type of surgery [7].

5.6   Postoperative Measures

Postoperative measures are crucial in the prevention and management of SSIs, playing a significant role in reducing the risk of complications and promoting optimal healing following surgery [51].

One important postoperative measure is the application of a dressing to cover the surgical wound. There are various types of wound dressings available, including hydrocolloid, hydrogel, fibrous hydrocolloid, polyurethane matrix hydrocolloid dressings, and vapor-permeable films [52]. Based on previous reviews [52], the WHO panel suggests not using advanced dressings over standard dressings on primarily closed surgical wounds for the purpose of preventing SSIs. This recommendation is made to ensure that resources are used effectively while still maintaining adequate wound care [7].

Special attention is also focused on the continuation of postoperative antibiotic prophylaxis. Current guidelines recommend a maximum duration of postoperative antibiotic prophylaxis of 24 h. However, emerging evidence suggests that a single preoperative dose (with additional intraoperative doses based on the duration of the operation) may be just as effective. Despite this, surgeons often continue administering antibiotics for several days after surgery as a routine practice [53, 54]. In line with guidelines from other organizations [5, 6, 36, 42], the WHO advises against prolonging the administration of antibiotics after the completion of the operation for the purpose of preventing SSIs [7].

The prophylactic use of drainage tubes after surgery has been a common practice. However, recent studies have raised doubts about the benefits of routine drainage [55, 56]. The WHO conducted a comprehensive systematic review to assess whether prolonged antibiotic prophylaxis with the presence of a wound drain is more effective in reducing the risk of SSIs compared to perioperative prophylaxis alone. Based on the findings of this review, the recommendation is that perioperative antibiotic prophylaxis should not be continued solely due to the presence of a wound drain. Instead, the decision to remove the drain should be based on clinical indications, although no specific evidence was found to recommend an optimal timing for drain removal [7].

5.7 Conclusion

This chapter has provided a comprehensive overview of existing IPC measures and guidelines in surgery, which are of utmost importance in ensuring patient safety and minimizing the risk of SSIs. Despite the availability of guidelines, adherence to best practices can vary, and certain recommendations may lack robust evidence. Furthermore, the applicability of these guidelines in diverse healthcare settings, especially resource-limited environments, needs to be considered.

There is a need for further research to address existing knowledge gaps and refine IPC practices in surgery. Studies should aim to provide stronger evidence for the effectiveness of specific interventions, optimize perioperative protocols, evaluate the impact of new technologies and approaches, and explore strategies for improving guideline adherence. Additionally, efforts should be directed towards enhancing surveillance systems and data collection to better understand the epidemiology and risk factors associated with SSIs. This will enable the development of targeted interventions and tailored approaches to IPC.

In conclusion, while significant progress has been made in IPC in surgery, ongoing research, collaboration among healthcare professionals, and continuous evaluation of practices are essential to further enhance patient outcomes and reduce the burden of SSIs. By applying evidence-based strategies, ensuring guideline adherence, and fostering a culture of infection prevention, healthcare providers can make a significant impact in minimizing the occurrence of SSIs and improving the overall quality of surgical care.

References

1. World Health Organization. Infection prevention and control. https://www.who.int/teams/integrated-health-services/infection-prevention-control. Accessed 16 Mar 2024.
2. Ban KA, Minei JP, Laronga C, et al. American College of Surgeons and Surgical Infection Society: surgical site infection guidelines, 2016 update. J Am Coll Surg. 2017;224(1):59–74.
3. Berríos-Torres SI, Umscheid CA, Bratzler DW, et al. Centers for Disease Control and Prevention guideline for the prevention of surgical site infection, 2017. JAMA Surg. 2017;152(8):784–91. Erratum in: JAMA Surg. 2017;152(8):803.

4. Borchardt RA, Tzizik D. Update on surgical site infections: the new CDC guidelines. JAAPA. 2018;31(4):52–4.
5. Leaper D, Burman-Roy S, Palanca A, et al. Prevention and treatment of surgical site infection: summary of NICE guidance. BMJ. 2008;337:a1924.
6. Scottish Antimicrobial Prescribing Group (SAPG). Good practice recommendations for surgical antibiotic prophylaxis in adults and children in NHS Scotland. https://www.sapg.scot/guidance-qi-tools/good-practice-recommendations/surgical-antibiotic-prophylaxis-in-adults-and-children-in-nhs-scotland/. Accessed 16 Mar 2024.
7. World Health Organization. Global guidelines for the prevention of surgical site infection. 2nd ed. Geneva: WHO; 2018. https://www.who.int/publications/i/item/9789241550475. Accessed 16 Mar 2024.
8. Storr J, Twyman A, Zingg W, et al. Core components for effective infection prevention and control programmes: new WHO evidence-based recommendations. Antimicrob Resist Infect Control. 2017;6:6.
9. World Health Organization. Core components for infection prevention and control programmes. Geneva: WHO; 2009. https://www.who.int/teams/integrated-health-services/infection-prevention-control/core-components. Accessed 16 Mar 2024.
10. Zingg W, Holmes A, Dettenkofer M, et al. Hospital organisation, management, and structure for prevention of health-care-associated infection: a systematic review and expert consensus. Lancet Infect Dis. 2015;15(2):212–24. Erratum in: Lancet Infect Dis. 2015;15(3):263.
11. German RR, Lee LM, Horan JM, et al. Updated guidelines for evaluating public health surveillance systems: recommendations from the Guidelines Working Group. MMWR Recomm Rep. 2001;50(RR-13):1–35; quiz CE1–7.
12. European Centre for Disease Prevention and Control. Surveillance of surgical site infections and prevention indicators in European hospitals—HAI-Net SSI protocol, version 2.2. Stockholm: ECDC; 2017. https://www.ecdc.europa.eu/sites/default/files/documents/HAI-Net-SSI-protocol-v2.2.pdf. Accessed 16 Mar 2024.
13. World Health Organization. Guidelines for safe surgery 2009: safe surgery saves lives. Geneva: WHO; 2009. https://www.who.int/publications/i/item/9789241598552. Accessed 16 Mar 2024.
14. Centers for Disease Control and Prevention. National Healthcare Safety Network (NHSN). https://www.cdc.gov/nhsn/index.html. Accessed 16 Mar 2024.
15. European Centre for Disease Prevention and Control. Healthcare-associated Infections Surveillance Network (HAI-Net): about the network. https://www.ecdc.europa.eu/en/about-us/partnerships-and-networks/disease-and-laboratory-networks/hai-net. Accessed 16 Mar 2024.
16. Rosenthal VD, Maki DG, Graves N. The International Nosocomial Infection Control Consortium (INICC): goals and objectives, description of surveillance methods, and operational activities. Am J Infect Control. 2008;36(9):e1–e12.
17. Gastmeier P, Schwab F, Sohr D, et al. Reproducibility of the surveillance effect to decrease nosocomial infection rates. Infect Control Hosp Epidemiol. 2009;30(10):993–9.
18. Gastmeier P, Sohr D, Rath A, et al. Repeated prevalence investigations on nosocomial infections for continuous surveillance. J Hosp Infect. 2000;45(1):47–53.
19. Barchitta M, Matranga D, Quattrocchi A, et al. Prevalence of surgical site infections before and after the implementation of a multimodal infection control programme. J Antimicrob Chemother. 2012;67(3):749–55.
20. Petherick ES, Dalton JE, Moore PJ, Cullum N. Methods for identifying surgical wound infection after discharge from hospital: a systematic review. BMC Infect Dis. 2006;6:170.
21. Dancer SJ. Controlling hospital-acquired infection: focus on the role of the environment and new technologies for decontamination. Clin Microbiol Rev. 2014;27(4):665–90.
22. NHS England. Health Technical Memorandum 03-01: specialised ventilation for healthcare buildings. 2021. https://www.england.nhs.uk/publication/specialised-ventilation-for-healthcare-buildings. Accessed 16 Mar 2024.
23. Anderson DJ, Podgorny K, Berríos-Torres SI, et al. Strategies to prevent surgical site infections in acute care hospitals: 2014 update. Infect Control Hosp Epidemiol. 2014;35(6):605–27.

24. Gastmeier P, Breier AC, Brandt C. Influence of laminar airflow on prosthetic joint infections: a systematic review. J Hosp Infect. 2012;81(2):73–8.
25. Sehulster L, Chinn RY, CDC, HICPAC. Guidelines for environmental infection control in health-care facilities. Recommendations of CDC and the Healthcare Infection Control Practices Advisory Committee (HICPAC). MMWR Recomm Rep. 2003;52(RR-10):1–42.
26. Mangram AJ, Horan TC, Pearson ML, et al. Guideline for prevention of surgical site infection, 1999. Centers for Disease Control and Prevention (CDC) Hospital Infection Control Practices Advisory Committee. Am J Infect Control. 1999;27(2):97–132; quiz 3–4; discussion 96.
27. World Health Organization and Pan American Health Organization. Decontamination and reprocessing of medical devices for health-care facilities. Geneva: WHO; 2016. https://www.who.int/publications/i/item/9789241549851. Accessed 16 Mar 2024.
28. Kovaleva J, Peters FT, van der Mei HC, Degener JE. Transmission of infection by flexible gastrointestinal endoscopy and bronchoscopy. Clin Microbiol Rev. 2013;26(2):231–54.
29. Derde LP, Dautzenberg MJ, Bonten MJ. Chlorhexidine body washing to control antimicrobial-resistant bacteria in intensive care units: a systematic review. Intensive Care Med. 2012;38(6):931–9.
30. Tanner J, Melen K. Preoperative hair removal to reduce surgical site infection. Cochrane Database Syst Rev. 2021;8(8):CD004122.
31. Seidelman JL, Baker AW, Lewis SS, et al. Surgical site infection trends in community hospitals from 2013 to 2018. Infect Control Hosp Epidemiol. 2023;44(4):610–5.
32. Kluytmans J, van Belkum A, Verbrugh H. Nasal carriage of Staphylococcus aureus: epidemiology, underlying mechanisms, and associated risks. Clin Microbiol Rev. 1997;10(3):505–20.
33. Schweizer M, Perencevich E, McDanel J, et al. Effectiveness of a bundled intervention of decolonization and prophylaxis to decrease Gram positive surgical site infections after cardiac or orthopedic surgery: systematic review and meta-analysis. BMJ. 2013;346:f2743.
34. Leaper DJ, Edmiston CE. World Health Organization: global guidelines for the prevention of surgical site infection. J Hosp Infect. 2017;95(2):135–6.
35. Bratzler DW, Dellinger EP, Olsen KM, et al. Clinical practice guidelines for antimicrobial prophylaxis in surgery. Am J Health Syst Pharm. 2013;70(3):195–283.
36. Joint Royal College of Surgeons in Ireland/Royal Colleges of Physicians of Ireland Working Group on Prevention of Surgical Site Infection. Preventing surgical site infections. Key recommendations for practice. Dublin: 2012.
37. McDonald M, Grabsch E, Marshall C, Forbes A. Single- versus multiple-dose antimicrobial prophylaxis for major surgery: a systematic review. Aust N Z J Surg. 1998;68(6):388–96.
38. European Centre for Disease Prevention and Control. Systematic review and evidence-based guidance on perioperative antibiotic prophylaxis. Stockholm: ECDC; 2013. https://www.ecdc.europa.eu/en/publications-data/systematic-review-and-evidence-based-guidance-perioperative-antibiotic. Accessed 16 Mar 2024.
39. Zimlichman E, Henderson D, Tamir O, et al. Health care-associated infections: a meta-analysis of costs and financial impact on the US health care system. JAMA Intern Med. 2013;173(22):2039–46.
40. Madrid E, Urrútia G, Roqué i Figuls M, et al. Active body surface warming systems for preventing complications caused by inadvertent perioperative hypothermia in adults. Cochrane Database Syst Rev. 2016;4(4):CD009016.
41. Wolfhagen N, Boldingh QJJ, Boermeester MA, de Jonge SW. Perioperative care bundles for the prevention of surgical-site infections: meta-analysis. Br J Surg. 2022;109(10):933–42.
42. High impact intervention: care bundle to prevent surgical site infection. London: Department of Health; 2011. https://webarchive.nationalarchives.gov.uk/ukgwa/20120118164404/http://hcai.dh.gov.uk/files/2011/03/2011-03-14-HII-Prevent-Surgical-Site-infection-FINAL.pdf. Accessed 16 Mar 2024.
43. Owens P, McHugh S, Clarke-Moloney M, et al. Improving surgical site infection prevention practices through a multifaceted educational intervention. Ir Med J. 2015;108(3):78–81.
44. Targeted literature review. What are the key infection prevention and control recommendations to inform a surgical site infection (SSI) prevention quality improvement tool? Version 4.0. ·

Edinburgh: Health Protection Scotland; 2018. https://www.nss.nhs.scot/media/2208/surgical-site-infection-ssi-prevention-quality-improvement-tool.pdf. Accessed 16 Mar 2024.

45. Culebras JM. Malnutrition in the twenty-first century: an epidemic affecting surgical outcome. Surg Infect (Larchmt). 2013;14(3):237–43.

46. Mainous MR, Deitch EA. Nutrition and infection. Surg Clin North Am. 1994;74(3):659–76.

47. Diana M, Hübner M, Eisenring MC, Zanetti G, Troillet N, Demartines N. Measures to prevent surgical site infections: what surgeons (should) do. World J Surg. 2011;35(2):280–8.

48. Stannard JP, Volgas DA, Stewart R, et al. Negative pressure wound therapy after severe open fractures: a prospective randomized study. J Orthop Trauma. 2009;23(8):552–7.

49. Roberts DJ, Zygun DA, Grendar J, et al. Negative-pressure wound therapy for critically ill adults with open abdominal wounds: a systematic review. J Trauma Acute Care Surg. 2012;73(3):629–39.

50. Stannard JP, Robinson JT, Anderson ER, et al. Negative pressure wound therapy to treat hematomas and surgical incisions following high-energy trauma. J Trauma. 2006;60(6):1301–6.

51. Seidelman JL, Mantyh CR, Anderson DJ. Surgical site infection prevention: a review. JAMA. 2023;329(3):244–52.

52. Dumville JC, Gray TA, Walter CJ, et al. Dressings for the prevention of surgical site infection. Cochrane Database Syst Rev. 2016;12(12):CD003091.

53. Kobayashi M, Takesue Y, Kitagawa Y, et al. Antimicrobial prophylaxis and colon preparation for colorectal surgery: results of a questionnaire survey of 721 certified institutions in Japan. Surg Today. 2011;41(10):1363–9.

54. Bratzler DW, Houck PM, Richards C, et al. Use of antimicrobial prophylaxis for major surgery: baseline results from the National Surgical Infection Prevention Project. Arch Surg. 2005;140(2):174–82.

55. Galandiuk S, Fazio VW. Postoperative irrigation-suction drainage after pelvic colonic surgery. A prospective randomized trial. Dis Colon Rectum. 1991;34(3):223–8.

56. Sagar PM, Couse N, Kerin M, et al. Randomized trial of drainage of colorectal anastomosis. Br J Surg. 1993;80(6):769–71.

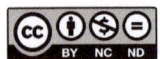

Multimodal Approach to Implement Infection Prevention and Control in Surgery

6

Maria Luisa Moro

6.1 Preventing Healthcare-Associated Infections

A significant proportion of healthcare-associated infections (HAIs) may be avoided adopting good clinical practices (GCPs) demonstrated to be effective in reducing the risk of cross transmission. Nearly 45 years ago, the pivotal study on the effectiveness of nosocomial infection control (SENIC) concluded that 30–35% of most HAIs were preventable with effective surveillance and control programs [1]. A much more recent systematic review, based on 144 studies published between 2005 and 2016, concluded that available evidence suggests a sustained potential for the significant reduction of HAI rates in the range of 35–55% associated with multifaceted interventions, irrespective of a country's income level [2]. Recently, the World Health Organization (WHO) estimated that 70% of HAI can be prevented by scaling up an array of effective infection prevention and control interventions [3].

However, several surveys and reports suggest that GCP recommended on the basis of scientific evidence are inconsistently and not uniformly adopted in daily practice. For example, before implementing change, the median compliance rate with hand washing was as low as 40% in 65 studies, mainly in intensive care units [4]. This, although the awareness of the importance of handwashing dates back to the 1800s and to Ignaz Philipp Semmelweis's discovery of the importance of hand hygiene. Similarly, in spite of universal agreement on several measure aimed at preventing surgical site infections (SSIs), three surveys conducted in Spain between 2016 and 2019, showed that the compliance with recommended measures for preventing SSIs was lower than 50% for several of the infection prevention measures surveyed, including management of body hair, appropriate surgical hand hygiene and decolonization of *S. aureus* with mupirocin [5].

M. L. Moro (✉)
Formerly at Regional Health and Social Care Agency, Emilia-Romagna Region, Bologna, Italy
e-mail: marialuisa.moro2022@outlook.it

6.2   Why Is It So Difficult to Translate Evidence into Practice?

In healthcare, one of the greatest challenges is how to introduce evidence and clinical guidelines into routine daily practice, i.e., translating research findings effectively and without undue delay from "bench to bedside". The problem is that, in particular contexts, multiple and often unpredictable interactions determine the success or failure of implementing changes.

Determinants for change may be categorized in factors relating to individual professionals, factors relating to social context and factors relating to organizational and economic context [6, 7] (Table 6.1).

Knowledge is fundamental for adopting GCPs and, consequently, education and training are the cornerstones for improving quality of care. However, behavior is strongly influenced not only by knowledge, but by attitudes, beliefs and personal traits as well. Pittet listed several examples of factors influencing individual levels relating to hand hygiene, e.g.: "Do nosocomial infections affect patient health? What is the impact of appropriate hand hygiene action to reduce the risk of cross-transmission? Would hand hygiene action damage my hands? Would it be time-consuming? Would it change my relationship with the patient? Would I be capable? How do others expect me to perform? How compliant with hand hygiene are my colleagues? Do I intend to clean my hands?" [7].

Healthcare professionals work in social, organizational and structural settings with specific factors that may support or impede change. People learn by observing others' actions and the results of those actions, as well as through role modelling. Moreover, the availability and easy access to rules and policies, as well as the

Table 6.1 Barriers to change: models and factors

Theories/models	Important determinants
Individual professionals	
– Cognitive	Mechanisms of thinking and deciding; perception of threat, balancing benefits and risks
– Educational	Learning needs
– Attitudinal	Expectancy/attitudes, perceived behavioral control/self-efficacy, social influences
– Motivational	Motivation to adopt the change
Social context	
– Social learning/ social network	Incentives, feedback, reinforcement, observed behavior of role models, values and culture of network, opinion of key people
– Patient influence	Perceived patient expectations and behavior
– Leadership	Leadership style, type of power, commitment of leader
Organizational and economic context	
– Organization	Innovativeness (incentives, feedback, behavior of role models, values and culture of network, opinion of key people), quality (culture, leadership), complexity (interactions between parts of a complex system), regulatory
– Resources/ economic	Availability of necessary staff and resources, reimbursement arrangements, rewards, incentives

Modified from [6]

availability of the necessary resources and of technical and informal structures helping to promote recommended behaviors, are among the institutional factors which influence the success or failure of introducing change.

A recent systematic review mapped barriers and enablers for adherence to surgical antimicrobial prophylaxis guidelines, concluding that an identification and understanding of these factors at a local level is required to develop tailored interventions to enhance guideline adherence [8]. A recent study showed that to influence infection control behaviors in surgery, interventions need to consider the social team structure and shared ownership of the clinical outcome in order to increase the awareness in specialties where SSIs are not seen as serious complications [9].

6.3   Which Strategies Are Effective in Achieving Change?

There is no evidence from systematic reviews that one of many approaches to change is superior in all situations; most are useful in some settings for some guidelines [10, 11]. Table 6.2 summarizes the principal interventions for changing behavior, but it is important to tailor each intervention to the specific local context [12, 13].

The most frequently studied interventions are those focused on individuals (educational meetings, audit and feedback, reminders, educational outreach visits and local opinion leaders). However, organizational interventions affect an individual's behavior and, to facilitate the adoption of new processes, adequate resources (time, people), strong management and leadership, and good communication systems are necessary.

According to a systematic review [14], multifaceted interventions (several elements or components implemented in an integrated way with the aim of improving an outcome and changing behavior), have a positive effect, particularly for more complex healthcare areas: interventions that link local opinion leaders, audit and feedback and reminders were the most effective strategies. Interventions where barriers to change were prospectively identified were more likely to be successful [15].

Table 6.2 Interventions that can be used to change health professionals' behavior

Interventions	Summary points
Individual level interventions	
– Educational materials	Modest effects but cheap and easy to implement. More effective if combined with other reinforcing strategies as part of a multifaceted intervention. Positive effect in more recent reviews
– Educational meetings	Smaller-scale interactive meetings are more effective than large scale didactic meetings
– Educational outreach visits	Effective but effect size varies depending on the clinical domain
– Opinion leaders	Mixed effect but some reviews reported positive effect when used as part of guideline implementation strategies
– Audit and feedback	Mixed effects, mainly small to moderate positive effects. Eleven reviews of multifaceted interventions found benefits to professional practice from audit and feedback

(continued)

Table 6.2 (continued)

Interventions	Summary points
– Reminders	Moderately effective in changing behavior, more effective if designed to specifically address barriers to change
– Patient-mediated interventions	Informing patients through mass media may be effective; providing educational materials for patients can help the implementation of guidelines; the impact of public reporting of clinician performance is unclear
Organizational level interventions	
– General points	Organizational changes can affect the individual's behavior; to facilitate adoption of new processes, organizations need adequate resources (time, people), strong management and leadership, and good systems of communication
– Specific changes	Changing professional roles can affect behavior; improving collaboration between professions may help the implementation of change
Multifaceted interventions	
	Multifaceted interventions can be more effective than single strategies, especially if barriers to change are identified and the choice of interventions is tailored to address these, and for more complex healthcare areas

Adapted from [12, 13]

6.4 Effectiveness of Implementing Preventive Strategies for Healthcare-Associated Infections

In the last decade, results from several systematic reviews have drawn a progressively clearer picture of the effectiveness of interventions aimed at implementing GCPs, through the adoption of implementation science. Multifaceted as well as monomodal interventions were evaluated.

Multimodal interventions intend to change behavior through implementation of several elements (e.g., system change, staff education, monitoring and feedback, reminders, culture change), using an integrated and multidisciplinary approach. Interventions can be supported by practical tools, including care bundles and checklists. Care bundles comprise a small set of evidence-based patient-focused practices (generally three to five), adherence to which is carefully monitored throughout the intervention. Care bundles are tools to guide the delivery of specific patient care practices, whereas multimodal interventions operate at organization level to change healthcare workers' behavior by implementing the abovementioned elements, and may include the use of care bundles [16].

The majority of implementation studies showed an increase in the compliance with the investigated practices and a decrease in HAI. Some reviews focused on general infection control practices in different settings [16–18]. Others investigated SSI, highlighting a significant increase in compliance with recommended practices and a decrease in SSI incidence: +95% compliance/−69% infections in 70 studies [19]; +100% compliance /−83% infections in 9 studies [20]; +19% to +92% compliance (depending on the number of bundle measures)/−44% infections in a meta-analysis of 35 studies (54,221 patients) [21]. Other studies looked at hand hygiene [22] central venous catheter infections [23], hospital pneumonia [24], urinary tract infections [25] or *Clostridioides difficile* infections [26], all testifying to a positive effect of these interventions.

6.5 How to Implement a Multifaceted Intervention

To effectively implement change, a systematic approach is needed, with accurate preparation and planning. The following steps are important: (1) formulating a concrete, attainable proposal, with clear targets; (2) assessing the actual performance; (3) analyzing what factors are stimulating or hampering the process of change, including resources, practicalities, as well as social and organizational context for the process of change; (4) selecting and developing a set of strategies for change; (5) developing and executing an implementation plan; (6) integrating the improvement within the normal practice routines; (7) evaluating and revising the plan [27].

Each intervention should engage the staff and leadership, be tailored to the local setting (investigating the actual performance and the most important barriers/enablers in that setting), conducted after a careful planning (including the selection of the most appropriate strategies), and complemented with a robust evaluation of the intervention outcome.

6.5.1 Engaging the Staff and the Leadership

It is crucial to understand how evidences can be integrated in the work process, given the context surrounding the work. Clinicians should be engaged to understand what is required to administer the intervention to patients, where defects can occur, or where the intervention is not implemented as intended [28]. Engaging frontline staff, largely by forming multidisciplinary teams, is a cornerstone of effective interventions. Team champions may be useful as well as partnering multidisciplinary teams with senior leaders and involving hospital leadership [19].

A recent guidance on the prevention of surgical site infections emphasizes the fundamental elements of accountability and engagement of various professionals for SSI prevention [29].

6.5.2 Assessing the Actual Performance and Analyzing Barriers/Enablers

To effectively promote the intervention is essential to identify and address local barriers to implementing the GCPs. The Agency for Healthcare Research and Quality has developed a specific tool—the BIM (Barrier Identification and Mitigation) tool—to assist in identifying barriers in promoting safe surgery [30]. It is also crucial to ensure that the health-care facility has the necessary infrastructure and resources in place for achieving change.

6.5.3 Selecting the Implementation Strategies

The WHO suggests five core components for multimodal interventions, for both hand hygiene compliance and SSI and has developed specific tools to support implementation [31, 32]: system change (i.e., ensuring that the necessary infrastructure is in place to allow health-care workers to practice change), training/education of healthcare workers, evaluation and feedback, reminders in the workplace to promote the desired actions, at the right time, and institutional safety climate (i.e., creating an environment and the perceptions that facilitate awareness-raising about patient safety issues while guaranteeing consideration of infection control improvement as a high priority at all levels).

The WHO model has similarities and relationship with another widely adopted implementation model known as the "Four ES". This model classifies strategies, as strategies aimed at engage (multidisciplinary network and strong leadership involvement); educate (various approaches to introduce evidence-based practices to clinicians and patients); execute (standardize interventions into simple tasks to facilitate uptake); and evaluate (assessing adherence with evidence-based interventions and patient outcomes, providing feedback of performance to providers) [19, 28]. This Four ES model has been recently incorporated by the Society of Hospital Epidemiologists of America in its guidance documents, to support efforts to accelerate improvement efforts.

6.5.4 Evaluating the Intervention

Regular monitoring and evaluation of recommended practices and procedures, infrastructures and available resources and supplies, and health worker knowledge and perception of the problem, coupled with timely feedback of SSI rates and risk factors for SSI, is vital if improvement is to be achieved. Evaluation and feedback should be seen as an essential step in identifying areas deserving major efforts and in feeding crucial information into the local action plan [32].

References

1. Haley RW, Culver DH, White JW, et al. The efficacy of infection surveillance and control programs in preventing nosocomial infections in US hospitals. Am J Epidemiol. 1985;121(2):182–205.
2. Schreiber PW, Sax H, Wolfensberger A, et al. The preventable proportion of healthcare-associated infections 2005–2016: systematic review and meta-analysis. Infect Control Hosp Epidemiol. 2018;39(11):1277–95.
3. World Health Organization. Global report on infection prevention and control. Geneva: WHO; 2022. https://www.who.int/publications/i/item/9789240051164. Accessed 16 Mar 2024.
4. Erasmus V, Daha TJ, Brug H, et al. Systematic review of studies on compliance with hand hygiene guidelines in hospital care. Infect Control Hosp Epidemiol. 2010;31(3):28–94.
5. Badia JM, Amillo Zaragüeta M, Rubio-Pérez I, et al. What have we learned from the surveys of the AEC, AECP and the Observatory of Infection in Surgery? Compliance with postoperative

infection prevention measures and comparison with the AEC recommendations. Cir Esp (Engl Ed). 2022;100(7):392–403.
6. Grol R, Wensing M. What drives change? Barriers to and incentives for achieving evidence-based practice. Med J Aust. 2004;180(S6):S57–60.
7. Pittet D. The Lowbury lecture: behaviour in infection control. J Hosp Infect. 2004;58(1):1–13.
8. Hassan S, Chan V, Stevens J, Stupans I. Factors that influence adherence to surgical antimicrobial prophylaxis (SAP) guidelines: a systematic review. Syst Rev. 2021;10(1):29.
9. Troughton R, Mariano V, Campbell A, et al. Understanding determinants of infection control practices in surgery: the role of shared ownership and team hierarchy. Antimicrob Resist Infect Control. 2019;8:116.
10. Grol R, Grimshaw J. From best evidence to best practice: effective implementation of change in patients' care. Lancet. 2003;362(9391):1225–30.
11. Grimshaw JM, Eccles MP. Is evidence-based implementation of evidence-based care possible? Med J Aust. 2004;180(S6):S50–1.
12. Robertson R, Jochelson K. Interventions that change clinician behaviour: mapping the literature. National Institute of Clinical Excellence (NICE); 2006.
13. Johnson MJ, May CR. Promoting professional behaviour change in healthcare: what interventions work, and why? A theory-led overview of systematic reviews. BMJ Open. 2015;5(9):e008592.
14. Medves J, Godfrey C, Turner C, et al. Systematic review of practice guideline dissemination and implementation strategies for healthcare teams and team-based practice. Int J Evid Based Healthc. 2010;8(2):79–89.
15. Chaillet N, Dubé E, Dugas M, et al. Evidence-based strategies for implementing guidelines in obstetrics: a systematic review. Obstet Gynecol. 2006;108(5):1234–45.
16. Price L, MacDonald J, Melone L, et al. Effectiveness of national and subnational infection prevention and control interventions in high-income and upper-middle-income countries: a systematic review. Lancet Infect Dis. 2018;18(5):e159–71.
17. Aboelela SW, Stone PW, Larson EL. Effectiveness of bundled behavioural interventions to control healthcare-associated infections: a systematic review of the literature. J Hosp Infect. 2007;66(2):101–8.
18. Edwards R, Charani E, Sevdalis N, et al. Optimisation of infection prevention and control in acute health care by use of behaviour change: a systematic review. Lancet Infect Dis. 2012;12(4):318–29.
19. Ariyo P, Zayed B, Riese V, et al. Implementation strategies to reduce surgical site infections: a systematic review. Infect Control Hosp Epidemiol. 2019;40(3):287–300.
20. Marche B, Neuwirth M, Kugler C, et al. Implementation methods of infection prevention measures in orthopedics and traumatology—a systematic review. Eur J Trauma Emerg Surg. 2021;47(4):1003–13. Erratum in: Eur J Trauma Emerg Surg. 2021;47(4):1015.
21. Pop-Vicas AE, Abad C, Baubie K, et al. Colorectal bundles for surgical site infection prevention: a systematic review and meta-analysis. Infect Control Hosp Epidemiol. 2020;41(7):805–12.
22. Price L, MacDonald J, Gozdzielewska L, et al. Interventions to improve healthcare workers' hand hygiene compliance: a systematic review of systematic reviews. Infect Control Hosp Epidemiol. 2018;39(12):1449–56.
23. Ista E, van der Hoven B, Kornelisse RF, et al. Effectiveness of insertion and maintenance bundles to prevent central-line-associated bloodstream infections in critically ill patients of all ages: a systematic review and meta-analysis. Lancet Infect Dis. 2016;16(6):724–34.
24. Mastrogianni M, Katsoulas T, Galanis P, et al. The impact of care bundles on ventilator-associated pneumonia (VAP) prevention in adult ICUs: a systematic review. Antibiotics (Basel). 2023;12(2):227.
25. Jones LF, Meyrick J, Bath J, et al. Effectiveness of behavioural interventions to reduce urinary tract infections and Escherichia coli bacteraemia for older adults across all care settings: a systematic review. J Hosp Infect. 2019;102(2):200–18.

26. Barker AK, Ngam C, Musuuza JS, et al. Reducing Clostridium difficile in the inpatient setting: a systematic review of the adherence to and effectiveness of C. difficile prevention bundles. Infect Control Hosp Epidemiol. 2017;38(6):639–50.
27. Wensing M, Grol R, Grimshaw JM. Improving patient care. The implementation of change in health care. 3rd ed. Oxford: John Wiley & Sons; 2020.
28. Pronovost PJ, Berenholtz SM, Needham DM. Translating evidence into practice: a model for large scale knowledge translation. BMJ. 2008;337:a1714.
29. Calderwood MS, Anderson DJ, Bratzler DW, et al. Strategies to prevent surgical site infections in acute-care hospitals: 2022 update. Infect Control Hosp Epidemiol. 2023;44(5):695–720.
30. Agency for Healthcare Research and Quality. Barrier identification and mitigation tool. Dec 2017. https://www.ahrq.gov/hai/tools/surgery/tools/surgical-complication-prevention/bim.html. Accessed 16 Mar 2024.
31. World Health Organization. A guide to the implementation of the WHO multimodal hand hygiene improvement strategy. Geneva: WHO; 2009. https://www.who.int/publications/i/item/a-guide-to-the-implementation-of-the-who-multimodal-hand-hygiene-improvement-strategy. Accessed 16 Mar 2024.
32. World Health Organization. Preventing surgical site infections: implementation approaches for evidence-based recommendations. Geneva: WHO; 2018. https://www.who.int/publications/i/item/9789241514385. Accessed 16 Mar 2024.

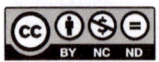

Antimicrobial Stewardship in Surgery

7

Nicola Petrosillo

7.1   Introduction

Healthcare-associated infections (HCAI) and antimicrobial resistance represent a major concern in public health. A point prevalence survey carried out in 2016–2017 in 1734 European hospitals assessed a prevalence of 5.9% HCAI among 325,737 inpatients. Methicillin resistance was reported in 31.0% of *Staphylococcus aureus* isolates with known antimicrobial susceptibility test results. Vancomycin resistance was reported in 11.4% of isolated enterococci and was considerably higher among *Enterococcus faecium* than *E. faecalis* (24.3% vs. 3.6%) [1].

Resistance to third-generation cephalosporins was reported in 34.7% of all Enterobacterales included for the selected antimicrobial resistance markers and was highest among *Klebsiella pneumoniae* and lowest for *Serratia* spp. Resistance to carbapenems was reported for 7.1% of all included Enterobacterales, also highest among *K. pneumoniae*, and in 32.2% of *Pseudomonas aeruginosa* isolates and 78.2% of *Acinetobacter baumannii* isolates [1].

In this survey, surgical site infections (SSIs) accounted for 18.3% of the total HCAI, representing the third most prevalent HCAI after lower respiratory tract and urinary tract infections. Gram-positive organisms were isolated in 46.5% of SSIs; among them, *S. aureus* (18.1%) and *Enterococcus* spp. (13.8%) were the most prevalent organisms. Gram-negative organisms accounted for 45.7% of isolates: among them, Enterobacterales and non-fermenting Gram-negatives accounted for 34.9% and 10.8% of the overall isolated organisms, respectively.

N. Petrosillo (✉)
Infection Prevention and Control/Infectious Disease Service, Fondazione Policlinico Universitario Campus Bio-Medico, Rome, Italy
e-mail: n.petrosillo@policlinicocampus.it

© The Author(s) 2025
S. Bartoli et al. (eds.), *Infections in Surgery*, Updates in Surgery,
https://doi.org/10.1007/978-3-031-60462-1_7

The most prevalent isolated organism in SSI was *S. aureus* (18.1%), followed by *Enterococcus* spp. (13.8%) and *Escherichia coli* (13.7%). Of note, fungi, mainly *Candida* spp. accounted for 4.3% of isolated organisms, while anaerobic bacteria, mainly *Bacteroides* spp., for 3.2% [1].

In this survey, about one-third of patients had at least one antimicrobial at the time of the survey, with an average of 1.37 agents per patient receiving antimicrobials. Of 102,089 patients on antimicrobials, 70.6% received one agent, 23.6% received two and 5.8% received three or more agents. Three patients received eight antimicrobial agents. The reason for antimicrobial prescription was treating an infection (70.6%), of which 70.1% for a community-acquired infection, 27.4% for a hospital infection and 2.7% for a long-term care facility-acquired infection.

Surgical antimicrobial prophylaxis (SAP) was the indication for 14.2% of prescriptions, and the prevalence of patients receiving surgical prophylaxis was 5.4%. The duration of prophylaxis was less than 1 day, 1 day, and more than 1 day in 26.8%, 19% and 54.3% of overall SAP, respectively [1].

Regarding the optimization of antimicrobial use, the definition of antimicrobial stewardship (AMS) consultant, which required mentioning of AMS activities as part of the job description, was not respected in 25% of hospitals reporting at least some full-time equivalent AMS consultant, and AMS activities were not part of any job description in 43% of hospitals [1].

7.2   Antimicrobial Stewardship: Definition and Aims

Probably the most accepted definition of antimicrobial stewardship comes from the Infectious Diseases Society of America (IDSA) that in 2012 reported that AMS "refers to coordinated interventions designed to improve and measure the appropriate use of antimicrobial agents by promoting the selection of the optimal antimicrobial drug regimen including dosing, duration of therapy and route of administration" [2].

As suggested by the ESGAP (European Society of Clinical Microbiology and Infectious Diseases Study Group for Antimicrobial stewardshiP), AMS can reasonably be defined as "a coherent set of actions which promote using antimicrobials responsibly" [3].

The main aim of AMS is to achieve the best clinical outcomes related to antibiotics; secondary objectives are to reduce adverse events, including allergy and diarrhea and to minimize the impact on antimicrobial resistance. As a consequence, excessive costs caused by the irrational use of antimicrobial drugs will decrease.

AMS in surgery includes the optimization of perioperative antibiotic prophylaxis for the prevention of SSIs and the proper use of antibiotics for infections related to surgery.

7.3 Perioperative Antibiotic Prophylaxis for Preventing Surgical Site Infections: An Antimicrobial Stewardship Priority

An SSI is defined as infection following an operation at an incision site or adjacent to the surgical incision [4]. SSIs occur in approximately 0.5–10.1% of cases, depending on the type of surgical procedure [5, 6] and are among the most prevalent healthcare-acquired infections [7].

Compared with patients without SSIs, those who develop them remain in the hospital approximately 7–11 days longer [8, 9]; one study involving 177,706 post-surgical patients reported that 78% were readmitted as a result of the infection [9].

Among the several measures to prevent SSI, one has a great value for antibiotic stewardship, i.e. perioperative antibiotic prophylaxis. The administration of antibiotic prophylaxis is recommended in all SSI prevention guidelines and has been reinforced by the World Health Organization (WHO) in its 2018 *Global Guidelines for the Prevention of Surgical Site Infection* [10].

Since the risk of infection increases as the time from antibiotic infusion to incision increases [11], antibiotics should be given within 60 min of the incision to maximize tissue concentration of the antibiotic [7]. However, since no significant difference in SSI rate was found when surgical antibiotic prophylaxis was given 120–60 vs. 60–0 min and 60–30 vs. 30–0 min, the WHO panel recommends the administration of surgical antibiotic prophylaxis within 120 min before incision, while considering the half-life of the antibiotic (strong recommendation, moderate quality of evidence) [10]. Moreover, the WHO also recommends to take into account the half-life of the administered antibiotics in order to establish the exact timing of administration within 120 min pre-incision.

Another recommendation is dosing antibiotics given for surgical prophylaxis according to the patient's weight to ensure adequate tissue concentrations and administering subsequent doses of antibiotics for lengthy procedures if excessive bleeding occurs [10].

Regarding the optimal duration of prophylactic antibiotics, prolonged antimicrobial prophylaxis is increasingly associated with patient harm, such as acute kidney injury [12].

In the light of the optimization of antimicrobial use, a systematic review of 28 randomized trials involving 9478 patients receiving either a single dose for prophylaxis or multiple doses concluded that additional doses did not result in any reduction in the risk of infection if the administration was prolonged [13]. An overall meta-analysis, which pooled 69 randomized controlled trials investigating the optimal duration of antibiotic prophylaxis in a variety of surgical procedures showed no benefit in terms of reducing the SSI incidence compared with a single dose of antibiotic prophylaxis [14].

Thus, the guidelines recommend stopping antibiotic prophylaxis when the surgical wound is closed.

Nevertheless, adherence to antimicrobial prophylaxis guidelines remains suboptimal, with values ranging from 25% to 80% [15–17]. In a recent retrospective cohort study of adults who underwent elective craniotomy, hip replacement, knee replacement, spinal procedure, or hernia repair in 2019–2020 at hospitals in the PINC AI (Premier) Healthcare Database, US, the authors evaluated adherence of prophylaxis regimens, with respect to antimicrobial agents endorsed in the American Society of Health-System Pharmacist guidelines, accounting for patient antibiotic allergy and methicillin-resistant *S. aureus* colonization status [15]. The PINC AI (Premier) Healthcare Database (by Premier Inc.) is an all-payer repository of claims and clinical data from more than 870 million US hospital encounters and includes approximately 1 of every 4 annual inpatient admissions [18]. In 825 hospitals enrolled, adherence to perioperative antibiotic prophylaxis was 59%: i.e., 308,760 out of 521,091 inpatient elective surgeries were adherent to prophylaxis guidelines.

The most common reason for nonadherence was unnecessary vancomycin use. In a post hoc analysis, controlling for patient age, comorbidities, other nephrotoxic agent use, and patient and procedure characteristics, patients receiving cefazolin plus vancomycin had 19% higher odds of acute kidney injury (AKI) compared with patients receiving cefazolin alone (adjusted odds ratio: 1.19; 95% confidence interval: 1.11–1.27; $p < 0.001$). Overall, this study found that approximately 40% of patients undergoing a major elective surgery did not receive guideline-adherent antimicrobial prophylaxis, largely due to unnecessary use of vancomycin, which independently increased the risk of AKI [15].

Another important point in proper perioperative antibiotic prophylaxis is the choice of the agent. For example, the most recommended agents for cardiac procedures belong to the class of cephalosporins [19]. A first-generation cephalosporin such as cefazolin is recommended, but in some hospitals also second-generation cephalosporins, with a higher impact on antimicrobial resistance, are given despite the recommendations. This is the case of a quality improvement study performed in a German tertiary care hospital that retrospectively studied 1029 patients who underwent cardiac surgery. Of these, 582 patients received cefuroxime and 447 patients received cefazolin following implementation of an AMS program following a revision of the standard for SAP. Overall, SSIs occurred in 37 (3.6%) of the cases, 20 (3.4%) in cefuroxime patients and 17 (3.8%) in cefazolin patients (*p* value = 0.7) [20].

An Italian study reported the results of an educational, participative, long-term continuing AMS intervention conducted between 2013 and 2019 in an Italian university hospital performing more than 40,000 surgical procedures per year. The authors collected and analyzed a total of 789 SAP prescriptions administered to 735 patients, of which 407 collected at baseline and 382 after the AMS intervention (2013 and 2019) [21]. The AMS intervention consisted of a series of structured audit meetings, attended by all professionals involved in perioperative antibiotic prophylaxis. Four months after the first survey period, appropriateness results were discussed with the prescribing personnel of each department, thus giving detailed feedback on perioperative antibiotic prophylaxis prescriptive performance.

In the study period, guideline adherence improved from 36.6% ($n = 149$) at baseline to 57.9% ($n = 221$) after the AMS intervention ($p < 0.0001$). A significant improvement ($p < 0.001$) was also detected for each appropriateness category: indication (from 58.5% to 93.2%), selection and dosing (from 58.5% to 80.6%), timing (from 92.4% to 97.6%), and duration (from 71% to 80.1%) [21].

7.4   Antimicrobial Prescriptions in Surgery: Room for Improvement

In addition to the fact that the inappropriate use of antibiotics generates worse clinical outcomes, their unnecessary use or misuse carries risks such as the emergence of antimicrobial resistance and adverse events, including the occurrence of *C. difficile* infections.

Identifying opportunities to safely reduce antibiotic prescribing in hospitals is necessary to enable prescribers and antibiotic stewardship teams to best focus their efforts to reduce antibiotic use.

Therefore, surgeons need to stay up to date not only with national and international consensus guidelines regarding the appropriate antibiotic prophylaxis for procedures they regularly perform, but also with recommendations and evidence on antibiotic treatment of the complications they most commonly encounter.

Clinical decision-making on antibiotic use (including empiric antibiotic selection), daily re-evaluation of the need for continued antibiotic therapy, and optimizing the duration of therapy should be basic expectations of surgical practice in the antibiotic-resistance era. Additionally, and most importantly, surgeons should be encouraged to seek consultation from their AMS team or infectious diseases consultant when questions arise [22].

The main opportunities for antibiotic stewardship in surgery, other than perioperative antibiotic prophylaxis, include:

– Decisions in empiric antibiotic treatment should be guided by the most likely pathogens, severity of illness of the patient, the likely source of the infection, and any additional patient-specific factors, including previous organisms identified from the patient and associated antibiotic susceptibility data in the last 6 months, antibiotic exposures within the past 30 days, and local susceptibility patterns for the most likely pathogens. Empiric decisions should be refined based on the identity and susceptibility profile of the pathogen [23].
– Limiting the duration of antibiotic treatment, especially when the source of infection is controlled. In 2015, in a randomized trial, Sawyer et al. demonstrated that in patients with intraabdominal infections who had undergone an adequate source-control procedure, the outcomes after fixed-duration antibiotic therapy (approximately 4 days) were similar to those after a longer course of antibiotics (approximately 8 days) that extended until after the resolution of physiological abnormalities [24]. The issue of the appropriate duration of antibiotic treatment in surgery remains unclear, and should be strictly related to the site of infection,

appropriate source control, antimicrobials targeted to the pathogens, pathophysiological status of the patient, and stability criteria.

- Source control, incision and drainage of superficial skin abscesses and opening of infected superficial SSIs is an effective treatment, for which antibiotic treatment could be shortened or, in some instances, avoided [22].
- Avoiding unnecessary antibiotics, such as in uncomplicated diverticulitis and asymptomatic bacteriuria. The surgeons should be aware that the use of antibiotics can trigger an intestinal dysbiosis leading to many pathological conditions including *C. difficile* infection.
- Facing complex infectious conditions, such as sepsis, as a team. Surgeons should not be alone in the management of complicated infections, such as intraabdominal infection with sepsis, but ideally inserted in a sepsis team together with intensive care physicians, medical physicians, pharmacists, clinical pharmacologists, clinical microbiologists and infectious diseases specialists, meeting periodically to reassess the response to the treatment [25].

7.5   Conclusion

Inappropriate antimicrobial use—including unnecessary use, overuse with respect to dosage or duration, and improper use of broad-spectrum antimicrobials—represents a challenge in surgical care. In an urgent call to action, AMS hand in hand with diagnostic and infection control stewardship may give opportunities for an improvement in the quality of care, contributing also to reduce the burden of antimicrobial resistance and adverse events, including *C. difficile* infection, in the healthcare setting [26].

References

1. European Centre for Disease Prevention and Control. Point prevalence survey of healthcare-associated infections and antimicrobial use in European acute care hospitals, 2016–2017. Stockholm: ECDC; 2023. https://www.ecdc.europa.eu/en/publications-data/point-prevalence-survey-healthcare-associated-infections-and-antimicrobial-use-5. Accessed 16 Mar 2024.
2. Policy statement on antimicrobial stewardship by the Society for Healthcare Epidemiology of America (SHEA), the Infectious Diseases Society of America (IDSA), and the Pediatric Infectious Diseases Society (PIDS). Infect Control Hosp Epidemiol. 2012;33(4):322–7.
3. Dyar OJ, Huttner B, Schouten J, Pulcini C, ESGAP (ESCMID Study Group for Antimicrobial stewardshiP). What is antimicrobial stewardship? Clin Microbiol Infect. 2017;23(11):793–8.
4. Centers for Disease Control and Prevention—National Healthcare Safety Network. Surgical site infection event. Jan 2023. https://www.cdc.gov/nhsn/pdfs/pscmanual/9pscssicurrent.pdf. Accessed 16 Mar 2024.
5. Dencker EE, Bonde A, Troelsen A, et al. Postoperative complications: an observational study of trends in the United States from 2012 to 2018. BMC Surg. 2021;21(1):393.
6. Seidelman JL, Baker AW, Lewis SS, et al. Surgical site infection trends in community hospitals from 2013 to 2018. Infect Control Hosp Epidemiol. 2023;44(4):610–5.

7. Seidelman JL, Mantyh CR, Anderson DJ. Surgical site infection prevention: a review. JAMA. 2023;329(3):244–52.
8. Zimlichman E, Henderson D, Tamir O, et al. Health care-associated infections: a meta-analysis of costs and financial impact on the US health care system. JAMA Intern Med. 2013;173(22):2039–46.
9. Anderson DJ, Kaye KS, Chen LF, et al. Clinical and financial outcomes due to methicillin resistant Staphylococcus aureus surgical site infection: a multi-center matched outcomes study. PLoS One. 2009;4(12):e8305.
10. World Health Organization. Global guidelines for the prevention of surgical site infection. 2nd ed. Geneva: WHO; 2018. https://www.who.int/publications/i/item/9789241550475. Accessed 16 Mar 2024.
11. Steinberg JP, Braun BI, Hellinger WC, et al. Timing of antimicrobial prophylaxis and the risk of surgical site infections: results from the trial to reduce antimicrobial prophylaxis errors. Ann Surg. 2009;250(1):10–6.
12. Branch-Elliman W, O'Brien W, Strymish J, et al. Association of duration and type of surgical prophylaxis with antimicrobial-associated adverse events. JAMA Surg. 2019;154(7):590–8.
13. McDonald M, Grabsch E, Marshall C, Forbes A. Single- versus multiple-dose antimicrobial prophylaxis for major surgery: a systematic review. Aust N Z J Surg. 1998;68(6):388–96.
14. Allegranzi B, Zayed B, Bischoff P, et al. New WHO recommendations on intraoperative and postoperative measures for surgical site infection prevention: an evidence-based global perspective. Lancet Infect Dis. 2016;16(12):e288–303.
15. Cabral SM, Harris AD, Cosgrove SE, et al. Adherence to antimicrobial prophylaxis guidelines for elective surgeries across 825 US hospitals, 2019–2020. Clin Infect Dis. 2023;76(12):2106–15.
16. Hassan S, Chan V, Stevens J, Stupans I. Factors that influence adherence to surgical antimicrobial prophylaxis (SAP) guidelines: a systematic review. Syst Rev. 2021;10(1):29.
17. Bardia A, Treggiari MM, Michel G, et al. Adherence to guidelines for the administration of intraoperative antibiotics in a nationwide US sample. JAMA Netw Open. 2021;4:e2137296.
18. PINC AI Applied Sciences. PINC AI healthcare database: data that informs and performs. 2022. Available at: https://offers.premierinc.com/Premier-Healthcare-Database-Whitepaper-LandingPage.html. Accessed 16 Mar 2024.
19. Bratzler DW, Dellinger EP, Olsen KM, et al. Clinical practice guidelines for antimicrobial prophylaxis in surgery. Am J Health Syst Pharm. 2013;70(3):195–283.
20. Surat G, Bernsen D, Schimmer C. Antimicrobial stewardship measures in cardiac surgery and its impact on surgical site infections. J Cardiothorac Surg. 2021;16(1):309.
21. Segala FV, Murri R, Taddei E, et al. Antibiotic appropriateness and adherence to local guidelines in perioperative prophylaxis: results from an antimicrobial stewardship intervention. Antimicrob Resist Infect Control. 2020;9(1):164.
22. Leeds IL, Fabrizio A, Cosgrove SE, Wick EC. Treating wisely: the surgeon's role in antibiotic stewardship. Ann Surg. 2017;265(5):871–3.
23. Tamma PD, Aitken SL, Bonomo RA, et al. Infectious Diseases Society of America 2022 guidance on the treatment of extended-spectrum β-lactamase producing Enterobacterales (ESBL-E), carbapenem-resistant Enterobacterales (CRE), and Pseudomonas aeruginosa with difficult-to-treat resistance (DTR-P, aeruginosa). Clin Infect Dis. 2022;75(2):187–212.
24. Sawyer RG, Claridge JA, Nathens AB, et al. Trial of short-course antimicrobial therapy for intraabdominal infection. N Engl J Med. 2015;372(21):1996–2005. Erratum in: N Engl J Med. 2018;378(7):686.
25. Vallicelli C, Santandrea G, Sartelli M, et al. Sepsis team organizational model to decrease mortality for intra-abdominal infections: is antibiotic stewardship enough? Antibiotics (Basel). 2022;11(11):1460.
26. Sartelli M, Duane TM, Catena F, et al. Antimicrobial stewardship: a call to action for surgeons. Surg Infect (Larchmt). 2016;17(6):625–31.

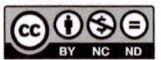

Principles for Correct Surgical Antibiotic Prophylaxis and Antibiotic Therapy

8

Massimo Sartelli, Guido Cesare Gesuelli, Rodolfo Scibè, Miriam Palmieri, and Walter Siquini

8.1   Introduction

Antibiotics have well-known benefits when prescribed appropriately. However, antibiotics are often misused, and giving them correctly is an integral part of good clinical practice [1]. Since the late 1920s, when Alexander Fleming discovered penicillin, antibiotics have revolutionized medicine and saved millions of lives each year [2].

Antibiotics are commonly used in acute care hospitals for the treatment of both community- and hospital-acquired infections and prophylaxis [1]. However, when they are prescribed incorrectly, antibiotics can offer little benefit to patients and, at the same time, potentially expose them and the community to risks for adverse effects [3]. Appropriate use of antibiotics means giving the right antibiotic to the right patient, at the right time, with the right dose via the right route of administration, and for the right duration [1].

Important considerations when prescribing antibiotics across the surgical pathway include understanding the difference between surgical prophylaxis, empiric therapy, and targeted therapy.

The term "antibiotic prophylaxis" refers to the administration of antibiotics to patients without signs of infection to prevent its occurrence. The term "empiric antibiotic therapy" refers to the administration of antibiotics to treat clinically suspected infections without antibiotic susceptibility test results, whereas the term "antibiotic targeted therapy" refers to the administration of antibiotics to treat microbiologically confirmed infections after receiving antibiotic susceptibility test results.

M. Sartelli (✉) · G. C. Gesuelli · R. Scibè · M. Palmieri · W. Siquini
Department of Surgery, Macerata Hospital, Macerata, Italy
e-mail: massimosartelli@gmail.com; gesuelli.guido@libero.it; rodolfo.scibe@virgilio.it; miriampalmieri92@gmail.com; walter.siquini@sanita.marche.it

© The Author(s) 2025
S. Bartoli et al. (eds.), *Infections in Surgery*, Updates in Surgery,
https://doi.org/10.1007/978-3-031-60462-1_8

63

Early detection of bacteria is required for optimally targeted treatment of infections. However, although great progress has been made in medical technology, the turnaround time, both for the detection and the characterization of bacteria, generally takes up to 24–72 h. As a consequence, clinicians start empiric antibiotic therapies, typically with broad-spectrum regimens, before a bacteriological diagnosis. Therefore, one of the major goals for prescribing antibiotics appropriately is to develop rapid diagnostic tests for identifying and characterizing bacteria as soon as possible.

Administering antibiotics is integral to the daily work of surgeons. It is important that surgeons know the minimal requirements, such as the antibiotic spectrum of activity and effective drug dosing. Without these minimal requirements, surgeons will increase the likelihood of treatment failures and adverse effects, including the selection of opportunistic infections such as *Clostridioides difficile* infection and the development of antimicrobial resistance.

8.2   Surgical Antibiotic Prophylaxis

Surgical antibiotic prophylaxis (SAP) refers to the use of antibiotics for the prevention of surgical site infections (SSIs). SAP is considered to be a key component of perioperative infection prevention measures [4]. Although compliance with the appropriate timing and spectrum of SAP has improved as a result of quality improvement initiatives, significant gaps remain in compliance with other aspects of SAP, such as the duration of postoperative antibiotics [4–6].

Given that approximately 15% of all antibiotics in hospitals are prescribed for SAP, antibiotic prescribing patterns can be a major driver for the development of opportunistic infections (such as *Clostridioides difficile* infections) and the selection of antibiotic-resistant bacteria, thus increasing healthcare costs.

Although appropriate SAP plays a pivotal role in reducing the rate of SSIs [1], antibiotics alone are unable to prevent SSIs and all infection prevention and control measures should always be considered.

Joint guidelines for SAP in surgical procedures were published in 2013 by the American Society of Health System Pharmacists, the Infectious Diseases Society of America, the Surgical Infection Society, and the Society for Healthcare Epidemiology of America [7]. These guidelines focus on the appropriate prescription of SAP. To be effective, SAP should have in vitro activity against the common organisms that cause SSIs after a specific surgical procedure. SSIs following clean procedures are usually due to Gram-positive cocci commensal skin flora, including *Staphylococcus aureus* or coagulase-negative staphylococci. Clean-contaminated (Class II) and contaminated (Class III) incisions may harbor various other bacteria depending on the flora of the specific mucosa incised, such as *Escherichia coli* or other Enterobacterales or Clostridiales.

An adequate concentration of the antibiotic should be present at the surgical site throughout the intervention, at (just before) the time of incision and for the duration of the procedure, that exceeds the minimum inhibitory concentration (MIC) for the likely bacteria associated with the intervention. The World Health Organization (WHO) global guidelines for the prevention of surgical site infections [8] recommend SAP administration prior to the surgical incision when indicated. These guidelines also recommend SAP administration within 120 min before the surgical incision, based on the half-life of the antibiotics. For the common antibiotics used, such as cefazolin, the ideal time is 30 min before the incision [9].

To be safe, SAP should have no or few adverse effects and should have the narrowest spectrum of activity necessary to prevent SSIs. SAP is suggested in surgical procedures associated with a high risk of SSIs, such as clean-contaminated surgical procedures. Although the incidence of SSIs is low for clean procedures where there is implanted foreign material (such as joint replacements), the guidelines suggest that the devastating consequences of a prosthetic-related SSI justify the use of SAP in these procedures. Therefore, the magnitude of both benefits and risks, in addition to the adverse effects of SAP, needs to be carefully considered in individual patients, depending on their risk factors and the planned procedure.

From a pharmacokinetic point of view, an additional intraoperative dose should be administered for procedures exceeding two half-lives of the antibiotic chosen [9] and again a third dose if that time interval is reached again later during a long operation. For operations with substantial blood loss (>1.5 L), the data are even less clear. In the case of cefazolin, which has a half-life of about 2 h, an additional intraoperative dose should be given after about 4 h. Otherwise, in the case of cefoxitin, which has a very short half-life of 40–60 min [8], a subsequent intraoperative dose should be administered after about 2 h.

The WHO global guidelines for the prevention of surgical site infections [8] recommend not prolonging the administration of SAP after surgical intervention to prevent SSIs. In 2020, a meta-analysis evaluating the effect of the postoperative continuation of SAP by de Jonge et al. [10] evaluated 83 relevant RCTs, of which 52 (19,273 subjects) were included in the primary meta-analysis. When best infection prevention practices were followed, the postoperative continuation of SAP did not provide any additional benefit in reducing SSIs.

8.3   Antibiotic Therapy

Antibiotic therapy is integral to the daily work of surgeons, but this therapy comes with competing responsibilities. On the one hand, surgeons should offer optimal therapy for the individual patient under their care by offering the antibiotic(s). On the other hand, they should preserve the efficacy of antibiotics and minimize the development of resistance and the selection of resistant bacteria.

Initial antibiotic therapy is typically empiric in nature because the patient needs immediate attention, and microbiological data (culture and susceptibility results) can require up to 24–72 h before they are available for a more detailed analysis.

Especially in critically ill patients, empiric therapy should be started immediately. Antibiotic therapy should be tailored to the individual patient, with narrower-spectrum agents used to manage community-acquired infections and broader-spectrum agents used for hospital-acquired infections.

In treating patients with hospital-acquired infections, the threat of antimicrobial resistance is one of the major challenges associated with antibiotic management. In the past few decades, an increased prevalence of surgical infections caused by antibiotic-resistant pathogens, including extended spectrum beta-lactamase (ESBL)-producing Enterobacterales, methicillin-resistant *Staphylococcus aureus* (MRSA), carbapenemase-resistant Enterobacterales (CRE) and non-fermenting Gram-negative bacteria—such as *Pseudomonas aeruginosa, Stenotrophomonas maltophilia*, and *Acinetobacter baumannii*— has been observed. Knowledge of local rates of resistance and the risk factors that suggest resistant bacteria should be involved as essential components of the clinical decision-making process when selecting which antibiotic(s) to use for empiric the treatment of these infections.

ESBL-producing Enterobacterales are now also present in community-acquired infections, and CRE are now endemic in the hospitals of many regions of the world and represent one of the most serious public health threats.

Obtaining microbiological cultures from blood, fluid, or tissue allows us:

- to expand the antibiotic regimen, if the initial choice is too narrow;
- to perform a de-escalation, if the empirical regimen is too broad.

Cultures should always be performed in patients with hospital-acquired infections or with community-acquired infections, in critically ill patients or in patients at risk for resistant bacteria.

When a bacterium is identified in clinical cultures, antimicrobial susceptibility testing should always be performed and reported, guiding antibiotic therapy.

One of the major goals for prescribing antibiotics appropriately is to develop rapid diagnostic tests for identifying and characterizing bacteria as soon as possible.

The timing, regimen, dose, route of administration, and duration of antibiotic therapy should always be optimized. In the context of a multidisciplinary approach, active communication with the infectious disease specialist and the microbiologist can improve appropriate antibiotic use and patient outcomes.

Knowledge of the pharmacokinetic and pharmacodynamic antibiotic properties of each antibiotic informs rational dosing. Optimal use of the pharmacokinetic/pharmacodynamic characteristics of antibiotic agents is important for obtaining good clinical outcomes and reducing resistance [11].

Dosing frequency is related to the concept of time-dependent versus concentration-dependent killing. Beta-lactams exhibit time-dependent activity and exert optimal bactericidal activity when drug concentrations are maintained above the MIC. Therefore, it is important that the serum concentration exceed the MIC for the appropriate duration of the dosing interval. Higher-frequency dosing, prolonged infusions, and continuous infusions have been utilized to achieve this effect. For beta-lactams, prolonged or continuous infusions have been advocated in order to maximize the time that the drug concentration exceeds the MIC, whereas high peak concentrations are not beneficial [11].

In patients with sepsis and septic shock, administering an optimal first dose is probably as important as the timing of administration. The optimal first dose, which could be described as a loading dose, is calculated from the volume of distribution (Vd) of the drug and the desired plasma concentration. The Vd of hydrophilic agents (such as beta-lactams and glycopeptides) in patients with sepsis and septic shock may be altered by changes in the permeability of the microvascular endothelium and consequent alterations in extracellular body water. This may lead to lower-than-expected plasma concentrations during the first day of therapy, resulting in suboptimal achievement of antibiotic levels. In the setting of alterations in the volume of distribution, loading doses of beta-lactams or glycopeptides are often required to maximize the pharmacodynamics ensuring optimal drug exposure to the infection site in patients with sepsis or septic shock.

The duration of antibiotic therapy should be shortened in patients with no signs of ongoing infection. The STOP-IT trial by Sawyer et al. [12] demonstrated that, in patients with complicated intra-abdominal infections when source-control procedures were adequate, the outcomes after approximately 4-day fixed-duration antibiotic therapy were similar to those after a longer course of antibiotics that extended until after the resolution of physiologic abnormalities.

Patients who have signs of ongoing infection or systemic illness beyond 5–7 days of antibiotic treatment benefit from further diagnostic investigations to determine whether an uncontrolled source of infection exists or the antibiotic regimen requires modification.

8.4 Conclusions

Appropriate use of antibiotics is an integral part of good clinical practice. This attitude maximizes the utility and therapeutic efficacy of treatment and minimizes the risks associated with opportunistic infections and the selection of resistant pathogens. The indiscriminate and excessive use of antibiotics appears to have been a significant factor in the emergence of resistant microorganisms in recent years.

In Table 8.1 the principles for appropriate surgical antibiotic prophylaxis and appropriate antibiotic therapy across the surgical pathway are illustrated.

Table 8.1 Principles of surgical antibiotic prophylaxis and antibiotic therapy

Surgical antibiotic prophylaxis (SAP)
- Antibiotics alone are unable to prevent surgical site infections. Strategies to prevent surgical site infections should always include attention to all measures of infection prevention and control
- SAP should be administered for operative procedures that have a high rate of postoperative surgical site infection, or when foreign material is implanted
- SAP should be bactericidal, nontoxic, and inexpensive. It should have in vitro activity against the common organisms that cause postoperative surgical site infection after a specific surgical procedure. Broad-spectrum antibiotics should be avoided for surgical prophylaxis
- SAP should be administered not more than 30–60 min before surgery for the common antibiotics used
- Therapeutic concentrations of antibiotics should be present in the tissue throughout the period that the wound is open. Additional antibiotic doses should be administered intraoperatively for procedures exceeding two half-lives of the antibiotic chosen and for operations with substantial blood loss (>1.5 L)
- Prolonged postoperative SAP should be always discouraged

Antibiotic therapy
- Antibiotics should be used after a treatable surgical infection has been recognized or if there is a high degree of suspicion of an infection
- The source of infection should always be identified and controlled as soon as possible
- Empiric antibiotic therapy should be started in patients with surgical infection, because microbiological data (culture and susceptibility results) may not be available for up to 24–72 h to guide targeted therapy
- Knowledge of local rates of resistance should be always an essential component of the determination of the empiric antibiotic regimen
- For patients with community-acquired infections, empiric agents with narrower spectra of activity are preferred
- For patients with hospital-acquired infections, antibiotic regimens with broader spectra of activity are preferred
- Targeted antibiotic therapy regimens should be adapted as soon as possible when culture and antibiotic susceptibility test results are available
- The antibiotic dose should be optimized to ensure that pharmacokinetic/pharmacodynamic targets are achieved. This involves prescribing an adequate dose, according to the most appropriate and right method and schedule to maximize the probability of target attainment
- The antibiotic therapy should be shortened in patients with no signs of ongoing infection
- Patients showing signs of sepsis beyond 5–7 days of antibiotic treatment should undergo aggressive diagnostic investigation to determine an ongoing uncontrolled source of infection

References

1. A global declaration on appropriate use of antimicrobial agents across the surgical pathway. Surg Infect (Larchmt). 2017;18(8):846–853.
2. Charani E, McKee M, Ahmad R, et al. Optimising antimicrobial use in humans—review of current evidence and an interdisciplinary consensus on key priorities for research. Lancet Reg Health Eur. 2021;7:100161.
3. Fridkin S, Baggs J, Fagan R, et al. Vital signs: improving antibiotic use among hospitalized patients. MMWR Morb Mortal Wkly Rep. 2014;63(9):194–200.

4. Sinha B, van Assen S, Friedrich AW. Important issues for perioperative systemic antimicrobial prophylaxis in surgery. Curr Opin Anaesthesiol. 2014;27(4):377–81.
5. Knox MC, Edye M. Educational antimicrobial stewardship intervention ineffective in changing surgical prophylactic antibiotic prescribing. Surg Infect (Larchmt). 2016;17(2):224–8.
6. Ozgun H, Ertugrul BM, Soyder A, et al. Peri-operative antibiotic prophylaxis: adherence to guidelines and effects of educational intervention. Int J Surg. 2010;8(2):159–63.
7. Bratzler DW, Dellinger EP, Olsen KM, et al. Clinical practice guidelines for antimicrobial prophylaxis in surgery. Surg Infect (Larchmt). 2013;14(1):73–156.
8. World Health Organization. Global guidelines for the prevention of surgical site infection. 2nd ed. Geneva: WHO; 2018. https://www.who.int/publications/i/item/9789241550475. Accessed 16 Mar 2024.
9. Sartelli M, Boermeester MA, Cainzos M, et al. Six long-standing questions about antibiotic prophylaxis in surgery. Antibiotics (Basel). 2023;12(5):908.
10. de Jonge SW, Boldingh QJJ, Solomkin JS, et al. Effect of postoperative continuation of antibiotic prophylaxis on the incidence of surgical site infection: a systematic review and meta-analysis. Lancet Infect Dis. 2020;20(10):1182–92.
11. Sartelli M, Weber DG, Ruppé E, et al. Antimicrobials: a global alliance for optimizing their rational use in intra-abdominal infections (AGORA). World J Emerg Surg. 2016;11:33. Erratum in: World J Emerg Surg. 2017;12:35.
12. Sawyer RG, Claridge JA, Nathens AB, et al. Trial of short-course antimicrobial therapy for intraabdominal infection. N Engl J Med. 2015;372(21):1996–2005. Erratum in: N Engl J Med. 2018;378(7):686.

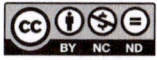

Microbiological Diagnosis in the Era of Antimicrobial Resistance

Gian Maria Rossolini, Alberto Antonelli, Angelo Galano, and Tommaso Giani

9.1   Introduction

Infections are a possible complication of surgery, with variable prevalence rates depending on the type of surgical intervention and epidemiological context [1, 2]. Most surgical infections are caused by bacteria or fungi colonizing the skin or mucosal surfaces of the patient, although cross-transmission of microbial pathogens via surgical procedures is also possible. The most common bacterial pathogens causing surgical infections are staphylococci (mostly *Staphylococcus aureus*), streptococci, enterococci, enterobacteria, Gram-negative non-fermenting bacilli (GNNFB) and anaerobes [2]. Fungal pathogens causing surgical infections are typically represented by *Candida albicans* and other *Candida* species [2].

Surgical infections are associated with a remarkable burden in terms of morbidity, mortality, and healthcare-associated costs [3]. In fact, the incidence of surgical site infection is considered among the indicators of healthcare quality by the WHO and other national and international agencies [1, 4]. The emergence and dissemination of antimicrobial resistance has compounded the burden of surgical infections by reducing treatment options and worsening outcomes [5].

Microbiological diagnosis provides an essential contribution for dealing with surgical infections, by identifying the causative pathogens and their antimicrobial susceptibility profiles, thus supporting antimicrobial stewardship. Knowledge about the nature of infecting pathogens may also be instrumental to rapidly enforce infection prevention and control (IPC) practices, to prevent dissemination

G. M. Rossolini (✉) · A. Antonelli · T. Giani
Department of Experimental and Clinical Medicine, University of Florence, and Microbiology and Virology Unit, Careggi University Hospital, Florence, Italy
e-mail: gianmaria.rossolini@unifi.it; alberto.antonelli@unifi.it; tommaso.giani@unifi.it

A. Galano
Microbiology and Virology Unit, Careggi University Hospital, Florence, Italy
e-mail: galanoa@aou-careggi.toscana.it

© The Author(s) 2025   71
S. Bartoli et al. (eds.), *Infections in Surgery*, Updates in Surgery,
https://doi.org/10.1007/978-3-031-60462-1_9

of microbial pathogens potentially causing surgical infections within the health-care setting. Finally, the cumulative information on infecting pathogens and their resistance profiles, derived from microbiological diagnosis, are important to define the local epidemiology of pathogens and antimicrobial susceptibility profiles, which is essential for the selection of the most appropriate empiric antimicrobial chemotherapy. The relevance of microbiological diagnosis has increased with the emergence and dissemination of antimicrobial resistance, which makes it more difficult to predict susceptibility on an empirical basis and complicates antimicrobial selection.

9.2   Challenging Resistant Pathogens in Surgical Infections and New Antimicrobial Options

Resistance issues are encountered among many of the pathogens responsible of surgical infections, which often exhibit multidrug-resistant (MDR) phenotypes (i.e., resistance to at least three different classes of antimicrobial agents).

Among Gram-positive pathogens, the major challenges are posed by methicillin-resistant *S. aureus* (MRSA), which was the first MDR pathogen spreading in hospital settings, and by vancomycin-resistant enterococci (VRE, usually *Enterococcus faecium*). Among Gram-negative pathogens, the major challenges are posed by members of the order Enterobacterales, by *Pseudomonas aeruginosa* and by *Acinetobacter baumannii* strains showing a difficult-to-treat resistance (DTR) phenotype, where DTR means resistance to the front-line anti-Gram-negative antibiotics including older β-lactamase-inhibitor combinations (e.g., amoxycillin-clavulanate and piperacillin-tazobactam), third- and fourth-generation cephalosporins, carbapenems, and fluoroquinolones, and possibly to additional agents like aminoglycosides and other non β-lactam antibiotics [6]. Gram-negatives showing DTR phenotypes typically carry a repertoire of antibiotic resistance determinants often including carbapenemases, which are β-lactamases capable of degrading most β-lactams including carbapenems [7].

The emergence and dissemination of DTR Gram-negatives, since the late 1990s, ignited the so-called antibiotic resistance crisis, a condition in which very limited or no options were left for treatment of infections caused by these pathogens, and the omen of going back to the pre-antibiotic era appeared to be eventually coming true [8]. Nowadays, several new antibiotics active against MDR pathogens are available in clinical practice, covering MRSA, VRE and also DTR Gram-negatives, with variable spectrum [9–11]. Under these circumstances, antimicrobial stewardship has become of the utmost importance in order to maximize the profit from the potential of the new antibiotics while reducing as much as possible the risk of resistance selection. In fact, the selective pressure generated by the use of novel antimicrobials has already shown the potential to select for resistance to these drugs, which is being increasingly reported [12–14].

9.3 The Contribution of Microbiological Diagnosis to Handling Infections Caused by Multidrug-Resistant Pathogens

Appropriate antimicrobial chemotherapy means prescribing an agent or a combination thereof that are active against the pathogen(s) responsible for the infection, with the overall narrowest spectrum to minimize collateral damage in terms of resistance selection. By providing information about the infecting pathogens and their antimicrobial susceptibility profiles, diagnostic microbiology contributes an essential input to the selection of appropriate antimicrobial chemotherapy.

The diagnostic microbiology workflow for bacterial and fungal infections is based on culturing clinical specimens on growth media to isolate the infecting pathogen(s) in pure cultures, which are then subjected to identification by biochemical assays or MALDI-ToF mass spectrometry, and to antimicrobial susceptibility testing by phenotypic antibiogram, which is an in vitro growth inhibition assay (Fig. 9.1).

This diagnostic workflow is universally adopted in microbiology laboratories, is well standardized and, so far, remains the standard-of-care for microbiological diagnosis and prediction of in vivo efficacy of antibiotics. In fact, clinical studies evaluating the efficacy of antimicrobial agents and outcomes in relation with appropriate/inappropriate selection of antimicrobial chemotherapy are overall based on the results of phenotypic antibiograms.

However, the conventional diagnostic workflow described above suffers from several drawbacks, including a relatively long time-to-results (TTR of 2–3 days at the shortest, depending on the type of clinical specimen) (Fig. 9.1), and a limited sensitivity for detection of some fastidious pathogens or in case of previous antibiotic exposure [15]. The long TTR mandates to start with empiric therapy, especially in severe infections, and possibly revise the regimen once results become available, with a higher risk of error in settings of higher resistance rates, where susceptibility of infecting pathogens is less predictable.

9.4 Novel Technologies for Microbiological Diagnosis

Recently, a growing number of novel technologies for diagnostic microbiology have been developed and introduced in clinical practice (Table 9.1) [16–30]. These novel technologies may offer some advantages vs. conventional diagnostics in terms of rapidity and/or sensitivity, which can overall improve handling of infected patients, including those with surgical infections.

Among the novel technologies for microbiological diagnosis, some measure antimicrobial susceptibility directly from positive blood cultures, in a shorter timeframe vs. conventional phenotypic antibiogram (i.e., 1–6 vs. 16–24 h), thus reducing the TTR of the conventional diagnostic workflow by 1–2 days. The technologies

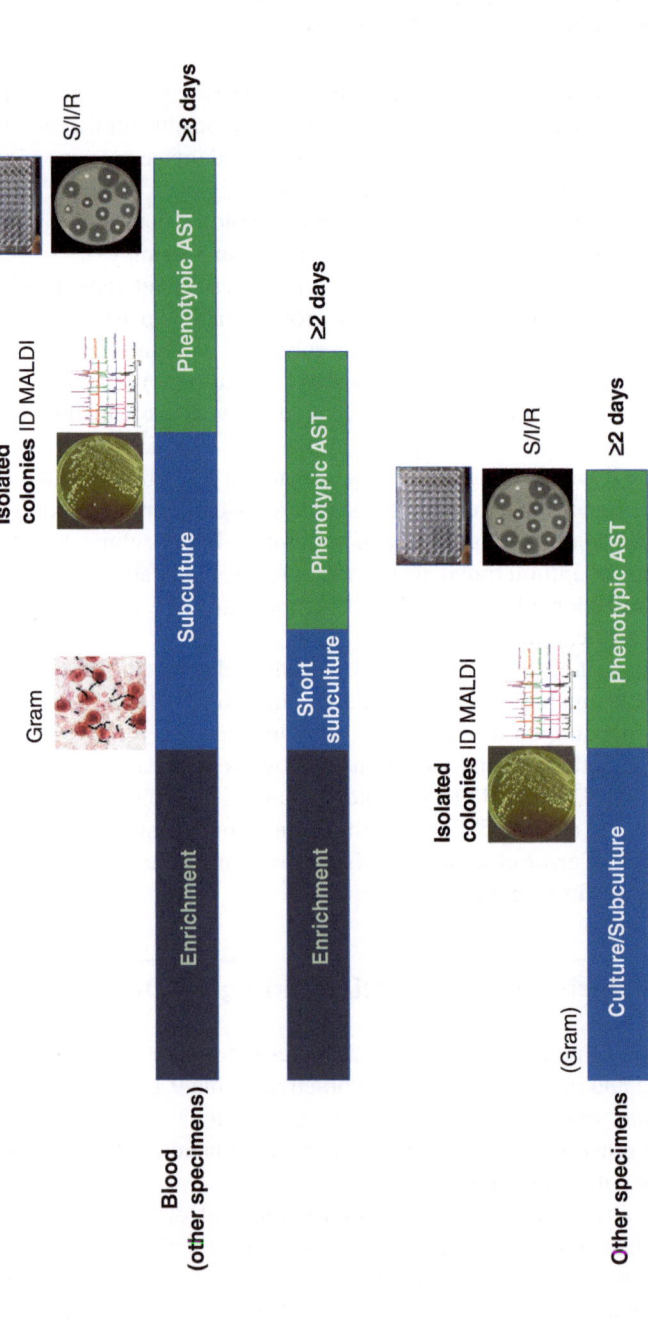

Fig. 9.1 The conventional culture-based workflow for microbiological diagnosis with clinical specimens. In the case of blood (and sometimes with other fluids), an enrichment step is necessary before culturing on solid media to obtain isolated colonies, which are required for identification of the pathogen by MALDI-ToF mass spectrometry and phenotypic AST (antimicrobial susceptibility testing) by disk diffusion or broth microdilution

Table 9.1 Novel systems for microbiological diagnosis

Novel diagnostic systems	Technology	Sample	Time to response	Results	References
Rapid phenotypic antibiogram	Time lapse microscopy	Positive blood culture	4–6.5 h	Susceptibility category/MIC value	[16–19]
	Volatile metabolites analysis		5–6.5 h		[20]
	Flow cytometry		2 h	Susceptibility category only[a]	[21]
Genotypic identification of pathogens and resistance mechanisms	Nucleic acid amplification technology (NAAT)	Whole blood	4–5 h	Species identification *or* resistance mechanisms detection	[22]
		Positive blood culture	1–5 h	Species identification *and* resistance mechanisms detection	[23, 24]
		Lower respiratory tract	1–5 h		[25, 26]
		Cerebrospinal fluid	1 h		[27]
		Synovial fluid	1 h		[28]
		Implant and tissue	4–5 h		[29]
		Intra-abdominal	4–5 h		[30]

MIC minimum inhibitory concentration

[a] Except for vancomycin and colistin MIC for *S. aureus* and Gram-negatives, respectively

for fast phenotypic antibiogram are based on advanced imaging of bacteria (e.g., by time-lapse microscopy), on the rapid analysis of metabolites produced by bacteria (metabolomics) exposed to different antimicrobial agents, or on flow cytometry analysis. Apart from rapidity, a major advantage of most of these technologies is that they return the same result as conventional antibiogram, i.e., minimum inhibitory concentration (MIC) values, that can be interpreted by clinical breakpoints (Table 9.1).

Other novel technologies for microbiological diagnosis are those based on the detection of specific DNA sequences in positive blood cultures or directly in clinical specimens. These technologies, also referred to as genotype-based diagnostic technologies, may have a number of advantages including: (1) rapidity, with a range of TTR of 1–6 h, while some of them can be used directly from clinical specimens; (2) high sensitivity, being culture-independent and exploiting signal amplification steps; and (3) in some cases (when functioning as standalone highly automated systems) the possibility of using them also in a near-patient mode, remotely controlled, which can be useful in settings with no laboratory facilities on-site.

Genotype-based diagnostic technologies not only provide microbial identification in a timely and sensitive manner, but can also detect genetic determinants for antimicrobial resistances of clinical relevance; for instance, *mec* genes associated with methicillin-resistance in *S. aureus*, *van* genes associated with vancomycin resistance in enterococci, and some β-lactamase genes encoding enzymes associated with resistance to third- and fourth-generation cephalosporins (extended-spectrum β-lactamases) and carbapenems (carbapenemases) [31]. Genotypic detection of resistance determinants can be very useful to rapidly inform about drugs that should or should not be used. For instance, genotypic detection of a *S. aureus* and of the cognate *mecA* gene in a clinical specimen obtained from a surgical infection suggests an MRSA infection and, consequently, the need for using antimicrobial chemotherapy with anti-MRSA coverage. On the other hand, genotypic detection of a *Klebsiella pneumoniae* and of a carbapenemases gene KPC in a clinical specimen suggests an infection by KPC-producing *K. pneumoniae* and, consequently, the need for using an antimicrobial regimen with anti-KPC coverage [32]; while genotypic detection of a *Pseudomonas aeruginosa* and of a VIM carbapenemases gene suggest an infection by *P. aeruginosa* producing the VIM metallo-enzyme and, consequently, the need for using an antimicrobial regimen with coverage for this type of resistant pathogen [33]. Genotypic detection of resistance determinants, also called genotypic antibiogram, returns actionable information as described in previous examples which, however, is notably different from that of conventional phenotypic antibiogram. In fact, the presence or absence of a resistance determinant does not inform about MIC values but only allows prediction of a likely resistance or susceptibility profile to some antimicrobial agents. For instance, detection of a *K. pneumoniae* and of a KPC carbapenemase gene allows us to predict a likely resistance to older β-lactams including amoxicillin-clavulanate, piperacillin-tazobactam, ceftolozane-tazobactam, third- and fourth-generation cephalosporins, and carbapenems, and a likely susceptibility to new BLICs with anti-KPC activity (e.g., ceftazidime-avibactam, meropenem-vaborbactam, and imipenem-relebactam) and cefiderocol, while no information is provided about susceptibility/resistance to non-β-lactam agents such as aminoglycosides, colistin, trimethoprim-sulfamethoxazole, and tigecycline. Despite these limitations, this is very valuable information to rapidly review empiric antimicrobial chemotherapy if anti-KPC coverage was initially not included. In fact, the rapid detection of carbapenemase genes has become a very valuable tool for guiding antimicrobial stewardship and the appropriate use of the novel antibiotics active against DTR Gram-negatives, since the profile of activity of these novel antibiotics differs, depending on the resistance determinant (Fig. 9.2). Clearly, this advantage is greater in settings where the prevalence of DTR Gram-negatives is expected to be higher, as in South-Eastern Europe, North Africa, Middle East, Latin America, and Southeast Asia [34, 35].

The genotypic detection of pathogens and of clinically relevant resistance genes is usually performed by the so-called molecular syndromic panels, which include panels of probes targeting the most common pathogens responsible for various infectious syndromes (e.g., bloodstream, lower respiratory tract, cerebrospinal fluid, implant and tissue, bone and joint, intra-abdominal and urinary tract infections) (Table 9.1) [31].

The genotypic approach to microbiological diagnosis has a number of advantages (see above) but also some limitations that should be acknowledged. A first limitation is represented by the fact that molecular syndromic panels only cover the

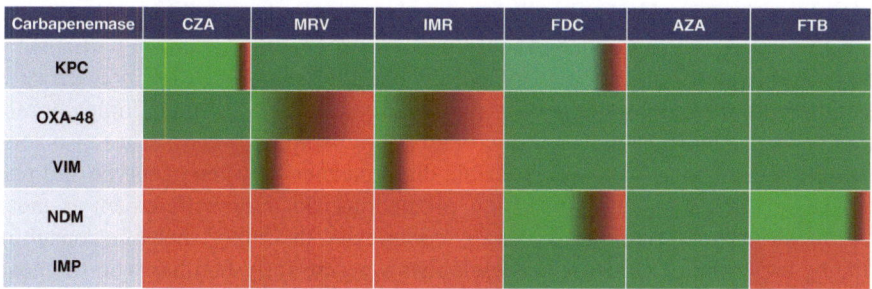

Fig. 9.2 Activity of novel antibiotics for Gram-negative DTR Enterobacterales producing different types of carbapenemases. Red color indicates resistance, green color indicates susceptibility. *AZA* aztreonam/avibactam, *CZA* ceftazidime/avibactam, *DTR* difficult-to-treat resistance, *FDC* cefiderocol, *FTB* cefepime/taniborbactam, *IMR* imipenem/relebactam, *MRV* meropenem/vaborbactam

most prevalent pathogens responsible for the various infectious syndromes: therefore, while a negative result is highly informative for excluding the presence of pathogens that are targeted by the panel, it is not informative about the presence or absence of pathogens that are not targeted by the panel. The same is also true for resistance genes, of which only some are targeted by the probes included in syndromic panels [30]. A second limitation is related with the possibility of discrepancies between genotype and phenotype. For instance, a resistance gene can be present but not expressed because of silencing due to various reasons (e.g., gene inactivation, lack of function of the promoter in a certain bacterial host): in these cases, prediction of resistance based on detection of the resistance gene may be misleading and can lead to overtreatment. On the other hand, detection of resistance genes by current syndromic panels does not allow us to quantitate the gene dosage, which can affect susceptibility to some agents. For example, an increased dosage of the KPC carbapenemase gene may lead to increased enzyme production and resistance to ceftazidime-avibactam and, possibly, also to meropenem-vaborbactam, imipenem-relebactam and cefiderocol. In this case, therefore, prediction of susceptibility to these drugs based on the results of genotypic antibiogram can be misleading.

Due to these limitations, microbiological diagnosis relying on genotypic testing still requires confirmation by the conventional phenotypic workflow. Possibly, in the future, the advent of new generations of genotypic diagnostic technologies based on WGS, shotgun metagenomics and transcriptomics will help to overcome these limitations.

9.5 Concluding Remarks

Microbiological diagnosis is essential for the properly handling of surgical infections. Nowadays, there are several novel technologies that may improve the quality and rapidity of the diagnostic workflow. Clinicians should be familiar with recent developments in the field of microbiological diagnosis to profit from their advantages but should also be aware of their limitations to avoid overinterpreting and to properly contextualize the results. Genotypic antibiogram, in particular, is becoming increasingly popular in settings characterized by a high prevalence of antimicrobial resistant pathogens to rapidly predict the presence of clinically relevant resistances and support antimicrobial stewardship. However, it has also some limitations, mostly related with possible discrepancies between genotype and phenotype, which can result in misleading predictions causing overtreatment or undertreatment. In this scenario of increasing complexity, the importance of a consulting role by experienced clinical microbiologists who are fully familiar with the novel diagnostic technologies should be emphasized.

References

1. World Health Organization. Global guidelines for the prevention of surgical site infection. 2nd ed. Geneva: WHO; 2018. https://www.who.int/publications/i/item/9789241550475. Accessed 16 Mar 2024.
2. European Centre for Disease Prevention and Control. Healthcare-associated infections: surgical site infections. In: ECDC, editor. Annual epidemiological report for 2018–2020. Stockholm: ECDC; 2023. https://www.ecdc.europa.eu/en/publications-data/healthcare-associated-infections-surgical-site-annual-2018-2020. Accessed 16 Mar 2024.
3. Paladini G, Elhadidy HSMA, Cornio AR, et al. Trends in mortality associated with surgical site infections: a cohort study in Italy, 2009–2019. Eur J Pub Health. 2022;32(Suppl 3):ckac129.595.
4. European Centre for Disease Prevention and Control. Directory of online resources for prevention and control of antimicrobial resistance (AMR) and healthcare-associated infections (HAI). https://www.ecdc.europa.eu/en/publications-data/directory-online-resources-prevention-and-control-antimicrobial-resistance-amr. Accessed 16 Mar 2024.
5. Sartelli M, Coccolini F, Kluger Y, et al. WSES/GAIS/SIS-E/WSIS/AAST global clinical pathways for patients with intra-abdominal infections. World J Emerg Surg. 2021;16(1):49.
6. Kadri SS, Adjemian J, Lai YL, et al. Difficult-to-treat resistance in Gram-negative bacteremia at 173 US hospitals: retrospective cohort analysis of prevalence, predictors, and outcome of resistance to all first-line agents. Clin Infect Dis. 2018;67(12):1803–14.
7. Bonomo RA, Burd EM, Conly J, et al. Carbapenemase-producing organisms: a global scourge. Clin Infect Dis. 2018;66(8):1290–7.
8. Bush K. Classification for β-lactamases: historical perspectives. Expert Rev Anti Infect Ther. 2023;21(5):513–22.
9. Bassetti M, Garau J. Current and future perspectives in the treatment of multidrug-resistant Gram-negative infections. J Antimicrob Chemother. 2021;76(Suppl 4):iv23–37.
10. Rodríguez-Baño J, Gutiérrez-Gutiérrez B, Machuca I, Pascual A. Treatment of infections caused by extended-spectrum-beta-lactamase-, AmpC-, and carbapenemase-producing Enterobacteriaceae. Clin Microbiol Rev. 2018;31(2):e00079–17.
11. Koulenti D, Xu E, Mok IYS, et al. Novel antibiotics for multidrug-resistant Gram-positive microorganisms. Microorganisms. 2019;7(8):270.
12. Coppi M, Antonelli A, Niccolai C, et al. Nosocomial outbreak by NDM-1-producing Klebsiella pneumoniae highly resistant to cefiderocol, Florence, Italy, August 2021 to June 2022. Euro Surveill. 2022;27(43):2200795.
13. Hobson CA, Pierrat G, Tenaillon O, et al. Klebsiella pneumoniae carbapenemase variants resistant to ceftazidime-avibactam: an evolutionary overview. Antimicrob Agents Chemother. 2022;66(9):e0044722.

14. Di Pilato V, Principe L, Andriani L, et al. Deciphering variable resistance to novel carbapenem-based β-lactamase inhibitor combinations in a multi-clonal outbreak caused by Klebsiella pneumoniae carbapenemase (KPC)-producing Klebsiella pneumoniae resistant to ceftazidime/avibactam. Clin Microbiol Infect. 2023;29(4):537.e1–8.
15. Arena F, Giani T, Pollini S, et al. Molecular antibiogram in diagnostic clinical microbiology: advantages and challenges. Future Microbiol. 2017;12:361–4.
16. Bhalodi AA, MacVane SH, Ford B, et al. Real-world impact of the Accelerate PhenoTest BC kit on patients with bloodstream infections in the improving outcomes and antimicrobial stewardship study: a quasiexperimental multicenter study. Clin Infect Dis. 2022;75(2):269–77.
17. Rosselin M, Prod'hom G, Greub G, Croxatto A. Performance evaluation of the Quantamatrix QMAC-dRAST system for rapid antibiotic susceptibility testing directly from blood cultures. Microorganisms. 2022;10(6):1212.
18. Malmberg C, Torpner J, Fernberg J, et al. Evaluation of the speed, accuracy and precision of the QuickMIC rapid antibiotic susceptibility testing assay with Gram-negative bacteria in a clinical setting. Front Cell Infect Microbiol. 2022;12:758262.
19. Göransson J, Sundqvist M, Ghaderi E, et al. Performance of a system for rapid phenotypic antimicrobial susceptibility testing of Gram-negative bacteria directly from positive blood culture bottles. Clin Microbiol. 2023;61(3):e0152522.
20. Tibbetts R, George S, Burwell R, et al. Performance of the reveal rapid antibiotic susceptibility testing system on Gram-negative blood cultures at a large urban hospital. J Clin Microbiol. 2022;60(6):e0009822.
21. Silva-Dias A, Pérez-Viso B, Martins-Oliveira I, et al. Evaluation of FASTinov ultrarapid flow cytometry antimicrobial susceptibility testing directly from positive blood cultures. J Clin Microbiol. 2021;59(10):e0054421.
22. Lucignano B, Cento V, Agosta M, et al. Effective rapid diagnosis of bacterial and fungal bloodstream infections by T2 magnetic resonance technology in the pediatric population. J Clin Microbiol. 2022;60(10):e0029222.
23. Caméléna F, Péan de Ponfilly G, Pailhoriès H, et al. Multicenter evaluation of the FilmArray blood culture identification 2 panel for pathogen detection in bloodstream infections. Microbiol Spectr. 2023;11(1):e0254722.
24. Burrack-Lange SC, Personne Y, Huber M, et al. Multicenter assessment of the rapid Unyvero blood culture molecular assay. J Med Microbiol. 2018;67(9):1294–301.
25. Webber DM, Wallace MA, Burnham C-AD, Anderson NW. Evaluation of the BioFire FilmArray Pneumonia Panel for detection of viral and bacterial pathogens in lower respiratory tract specimens in the setting of a tertiary care academic medical center. J Clin Microbiol. 2020;58(7):e00343–20.
26. Klein M, Bacher J, Barth S, et al. Multicenter evaluation of the Unyvero platform for testing bronchoalveolar lavage fluid. J Clin Microbiol. 2021;59(3):e02497–20.
27. Trujillo-Gómez J, Tsokani S, Arango-Ferreira C, et al. Biofire FilmArray Meningitis/Encephalitis panel for the aetiological diagnosis of central nervous system infections: a systematic review and diagnostic test accuracy meta-analysis. EClinicalMedicine. 2022;44:101275.
28. Saeed K, Ahmad-Saeed N, Annett R, et al. A multicentre evaluation and expert recommendations of use of the newly developed BioFire Joint Infection polymerase chain reaction panel. Eur J Clin Microbiol Infect Dis. 2023;42(2):169–76.
29. Papan C, Meyer-Buehn M, Laniado G, Huebner J. Evaluation of the multiplex PCR based assay Unyvero implant and tissue infection application for pathogen and antibiotic resistance gene detection in children and neonates. Infection. 2019;47(2):195–200.
30. Ciesielczuk H, Wilks M, Castelain S, et al. Multicenter performance evaluation of the Unyvero IAI cartridge for detection of intra-abdominal infections. Eur J Clin Microbiol Infect Dis. 2018;37(11):2107–15.
31. Relich RF, Abbott AN. Syndromic and point-of-care molecular testing. Clin Lab Med. 2022;42(4):507–31.
32. Bassetti M, Kanj SS, Kiratisin P, et al. Early appropriate diagnostics and treatment of MDR Gram-negative infections. JAC Antimicrob Resist. 2022;4(5):dlac089.

33. Losito AR, Raffaelli F, Del Giacomo P, Tumbarello M. New drugs for the treatment of Pseudomonas aeruginosa infections with limited treatment options: a narrative review. Antibiotics (Basel). 2022;11(5):579.
34. Antimicrobial Resistance Collaborators. Global burden of bacterial antimicrobial resistance in 2019: a systematic analysis. Lancet. 2022;399(10325):629–55. Erratum in: Lancet. 2022;400(10358):1102.
35. Oldenkamp R, Schultsz C, Mancini E, Cappuccio A. Filling the gaps in the global prevalence map of clinical antimicrobial resistance. Proc Natl Acad Sci U S A. 2021;118(1):e2013515118. Erratum in: Proc Natl Acad Sci U S A. 2021;118(42):e2116827118.

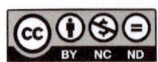

Infection Prevention and Control in Acute Care Surgery

10

Giorgia Santandrea, Carlo Vallicelli, Massimo Sartelli, Federico Coccolini, Luca Ansaloni, Vanni Agnoletti, and Fausto Catena

10.1 Classification and Diagnosis of Intra-Abdominal Infections

In the evaluation of intra-abdominal infections (IAIs) there are several parameters to consider, such as anatomical extent, presumed pathogens involved, local antibiotic resistance patterns and the patient's clinical condition. IAIs can be classified as uncomplicated, which involve a single organ and do not extend to the peritoneum, or complicated, when the infection proceeds beyond the organ into the peritoneum, causing localized or diffuse peritonitis [1]. Peritonitis, depending on the underlying pathology, can be sterile or infectious.

G. Santandrea · C. Vallicelli · F. Catena (✉)
Emergency and Trauma Surgery Department, Bufalini Hospital, Cesena, Italy
e-mail: giorgia.santandrea@auslromagna.it; carlo.vallicelli@auslromagna.it; fausto.catena@auslromagna.it

M. Sartelli
Department of Surgery, Macerata Hospital, Macerata, Italy
e-mail: massimosartelli@gmail.com

F. Coccolini
General, Trauma and Emergency Surgery Department, Pisa University Hospital, Pisa, Italy
e-mail: federico.coccolini@gmail.com

L. Ansaloni
General, Emergency and Trauma Surgery Department, Policlinico San Matteo Hospital, Pavia, Italy
e-mail: aiace63@gmail.com

V. Agnoletti
Intensive Care Unit, Bufalini Hospital, Cesena, Italy
e-mail: vanni.agnoletti@auslromagna.it

S. Bartoli et al. (eds.), *Infections in Surgery*, Updates in Surgery,
https://doi.org/10.1007/978-3-031-60462-1_10

Infectious peritonitis is classified into [2]:

- *primary*: diffuse bacterial infection without loss of integrity of the gastrointestinal tract (typical of patients with cirrhotic ascites or patients undergoing peritoneal dialysis); it usually requires no surgical treatment;
- *secondary* (the most common form), due to loss of integrity of the gastrointestinal tract;
- *tertiary*: recurrent peritoneal infection which occurs more than 48 h after apparently successful and adequate surgical source control of secondary peritonitis (usually associated with multidrug-resistant organisms, common in immunocompromised patients, associated with high morbidity and mortality).

Moreover, infections in emergency surgery can be classified into community-acquired and healthcare-associated abdominal infections, infections occurring in a patient during the process of care in a hospital or other healthcare facility which were not present or incubating at the time of admission. This differentiation is useful to define the presumed resistance patterns and identify patients with increased likelihood of infections caused by multidrug-resistant microorganisms [3, 4]. Healthcare-associated infections are: surgical site infections, catheter-associated urinary infections, hospital-acquired pneumonia, ventilator-associated pneumonia, central venous catheter-associated bloodstream infections, and *Clostridioides difficile* infections. Patients with healthcare-associated infections are more likely to have a longer hospital stay, require second-line or broader-spectrum and more expansive antimicrobials and place greater demands on the health system. The application of appropriate prevention and control strategies by the healthcare workers can reduce the risk of healthcare-associated infections. Good clinical practice is based on infection prevention and control, adequate source control and antimicrobial stewardship.

10.2   Infection Prevention and Control

Prevention of surgical site infection comprises:

- patient preoperative bathing or showering;
- appropriate surgical antibiotic prophylaxis;
- avoiding hair removal;
- correct surgical hand scrubbing/preparation. Using gloves does not replace the need for cleaning hands;
- correct skin antiseptic preparation.

Early clinical evaluation is essential in the diagnostic process, in order to optimize diagnostic testing and establish the proper therapeutic plan. The typical presentation consists in abdominal pain and signs of local and systemic inflammation (pain, tenderness, fever, tachycardia and/or tachypnea); signs such as oliguria, acute alteration of mental status, lactic acidosis are indicative of organ failure sustained by hypotension and hypoperfusion. Physical evaluation may help in the differential diagnosis to direct decisions about diagnostic testing (ultrasound, computed tomography, magnetic resonance imaging) and patient management [5]. Prognostic scores may be useful in clinical practice to assess the severity and the prognosis of the disease and help in selecting treatment and patient management options. Scoring systems can be divided into two groups:

- *general organ failure severity (ICU) scores*: these assess various organ systems for the presence of dysfunction and are used in sepsis and other causes of multi-organ failure (examples are the APACHE II score, SAPS score [6], and SOFA score [7]);
- *peritonitis-specific (surgical) scores*: calculated before and during surgery, these often include characteristics of the peritoneal contamination (examples are: the P-Possum score, MPI score, PIA score [8], and the WSES complicated IAI score from the WISS study [9]).

10.3 Source Control

The majority of patients with IAIs should undergo an urgent source control procedure, to eliminate the source of infection and control contamination. It should be performed as soon as possible in patients with diffuse peritonitis, but it could be delayed not more than 24 h in patients with a localized infection if appropriate antimicrobial therapy is given [5]. Source control can be delayed in severely ill patients. Operative intervention remains the treatment of choice in IAIs. It includes percutaneous drainage or surgical treatment. Well-localized fluid collections of adequate density and consistency can be drained percutaneously [10, 11]. Surgical source control comprises resection or suture of diseased viscus, removal of the infected organ, debridement of necrotic tissue, resection of ischemic bowel, repair/resection of traumatic lesions. Laparoscopic lavage in complicated acute diverticulitis is debated and its utility is not demonstrated [12]: in the majority of cases, in patients with complicated acute diverticulitis, percutaneous drainage of abscesses or surgical resection are preferred. Highly selected patients with complicated diverticulitis, including those with abscesses less than 4 cm, a periappendicular mass or a perforated peptic ulcer can be managed without source control if responding to antimicrobial therapy and other supportive measures. Abscesses may be treated by intravenous antibiotics alone or with percutaneous drainage, depending on the size (a maximum diameter of 3–6 cm is usually accepted for antibiotic treatment) [13, 14]. Antibiotics alone may be used in patients with early, non-perforated appendicitis [15]; also in patients with complicated appendicitis (abscess or phlegmons) non-operative treatment can be tried [16, 17].

Damage control surgery may be an option in selected physiologically deranged septic patients, in order to allow early draining of any residual infection and control any persistent source of infection, postponing definitive intervention until the patient is hemodynamically stable [18]. Application of negative pressure wound therapy devices can be useful to decrease the time to definitive abdominal closure, reducing the complications related to open abdomen [19, 20]. Prolonged negative pressure increases the risk of enteric fistulae [1].

10.4 Principles of Antimicrobial Prophylaxis and Therapy

With regard to antibiotic prophylaxis, it is possible to summarize some fundamental strategies:

- Antibiotics alone are unable to prevent surgical site infections, but it is important to combine their use with infection control and prevention measures.
- Antibiotic prophylaxis should be administered for operative procedures that have a high rate of postoperative surgical site infection, or when foreign materials are implanted.
- Antibiotics should be effective against the aerobic and anaerobic pathogens more likely to contaminate through surgical sites (Gram-positive skin commensals or normal flora colonizing the incised mucosae).
- Administration of the first dose of antibiotics beginning within 30–60 min before surgical incision is recommended for most antibiotics to ensure adequate serum and tissue concentration during the period of potential contamination.
- A single dose is generally sufficient. Additional antibiotic doses should be administered intraoperatively for procedures longer than 2–4 h, or with associated significant blood-loss (more than 1.5 L).
- There is no evidence to support the use of postoperative antibiotic prophylaxis.

Antibiotics are often used inappropriately. In the past two decades the incidence of infections caused by multidrug-resistant microorganisms has risen dramatically across surgical departments worldwide, correlating with escalating levels of antibiotic exposure. Appropriate use of antibiotics is important to limit antimicrobial resistance, to decrease *C. difficile* infections, to improve patient outcomes, and to reduce adverse antibiotic events. Empiric antimicrobial therapy should be based on local epidemiology, patient risk factors, clinical severity of the infection and infection source. The principles of antibiotic therapy should be defined according to the most frequently isolated microbes, taking into consideration the local trend of antibiotic resistance. For patients with community-acquired IAIs, agents with narrower spectrum of activity should be suggested; by contrast, in patients with healthcare-associated IAIs, broader-spectrum antimicrobials are preferred [1]. Usually, it is important to take into account corticosteroid use, organ transplantation, pulmonary or hepatic disease, and previous antimicrobial therapy [21]. Previous antimicrobial therapy is the most important factor for resistant pathogens [4]. An ineffective or inadequate antimicrobial regimen is one of the variables most frequently associated with negative outcomes in critically ill patients. Intravenous antibiotics should be administered as soon as possible and in any case within the first hour of onset of sepsis, using the broad-spectrum agents with adequate penetration of the presumed site of infection [22–24].

The correct dose and correct administration of antimicrobials should include:

- *Loading dose when indicated*: a higher than standard loading dose of hydrophilic agents, such as β-lactams, should be administered to obtain optimal exposure at the infection site [25]; missing of loading dose results in an underexposure to hydrophilic antibiotics that may be critical for the patient [26, 27]. Once the appropriate loading dose is administered, daily reassessment of the antimicrobial regimen should be done.
- *Extended or prolonged infusion for β-lactam antibiotics*: some antibiotics have time-dependent activity and their action is optimal when drug concentrations are maintained above the minimum inhibitory concentration (MIC), whereas high peak concentrations are not beneficial. This is the reason why some antibiotics, such as β-lactams have better action if administered with prolonged or continuous infusion. On the other hand, for antibiotics with concentration-dependent activity, such as aminoglycosides, the use of higher doses at extended intervals is recommended [28].
- *Peritoneal distribution*: the concentration gradient between the plasma and the peritoneal space may be relevant in the case of multidrug resistant microorganisms. Moreover, some disease and drug-related factors contribute to differential tissue distribution [29].

Intraperitoneal specimens for microbiological evaluation from the site of infection are always recommended for patients with healthcare-associated IAI and for those with community-acquired IAI at risk for resistant pathogens because of previous antibiotic therapy, and in critically ill patients. Appropriate intraperitoneal specimen is peritoneal fluid or tissue collected from the site of infection. Once the results of microbiological testing are available, the patient should be reassessed, as the results provide the opportunity to expand the antimicrobial regimen if the initial choice was too narrow, but also allow de-escalation if the empirical regimen was too broad [1].

Optimal duration of antimicrobial therapy depends on the kind of IAI:

- Uncomplicated acute cholecystitis and uncomplicated surgically treated acute appendicitis do not need antibiotic therapy, because the source of infection has been completely removed.
- In patients with IAI who are not severely ill and when source control is adequate, a short-course (3–5 days) antibiotic therapy is suggested.
- In patients with ongoing or persistent IAI, the decision to continue, revise or stop antimicrobial therapy should be based on clinical judgment and laboratory information. Procalcitonin has been suggested as a useful marker to guide therapeutic decision-making in the management of sepsis, and it may be helpful to determine the timing and appropriateness of escalation of antimicrobial therapy [30].
- If the patient is critically ill, the treatment duration can be deferred until after a careful multidisciplinary evaluation. Inadequate source control and

inappropriate antibiotics are determinants of mortality in patients with IAI and associated bacteremia. Principal determinants of antibiotic choice in critically ill patients are based on three main parameters: severity of illness, local ecology and host risk factors. Previous antibiotic use is associated with a higher development of multidrug-resistant organisms. Broad spectrum antibiotic therapy and previous antibiotic administration (within the first hour of recognition of severe sepsis) are recommended. Factors independently associated with in-hospital mortality are septic shock, high SOFA score and inadequate empirical therapy. De-escalation therapy once the antimicrobial sample is available is a protective factor against selection of multidrug-resistant microorganisms [1].

The presence of *Candida* spp. in the peritoneal samples is a factor of poor prognosis [31]. In community-acquired infections, the role of *Candida* spp. in the prognosis is difficult to demonstrate, while in healthcare-associated peritonitis it is associated with increased mortality [32]. Situations that justify an empirical antifungal therapy are patients with septic shock in community-acquired infections or patients with postoperative infections. The need for an early adequate systemic antifungal therapy in *Candida* peritonitis is based on the assumption that delayed antifungal therapy is associated with poorer outcomes [33, 34]. Optimal duration of treatment is not established: based on the high rates of recurrence and relapse in *Candida* IAIs, a duration of 2–3 weeks is recommended [35].

A rational use of antibiotics is important in order to prevent emergence of multidrug-resistant bacteria, above all in intensive care units. Antibiotic stewardship programs can both optimize the treatment of infection and reduce adverse events associated with antibiotic use. Their aims are to educate healthcare workers, limit antimicrobial resistance, decrease adverse antibiotic events, reduce healthcare costs, decrease *C. difficile* infections, reduce inappropriate antibiotics use, improve patient outcome, and increase adherence to guidelines [22]. Interventions to improve antibiotic prescribing practices should be directed at patient level (including clinical severity, epidemiological exposures, comorbidities, prior antibiotic exposure, prior infection, infection source), and hospital level (presence of in-hospital stewardship programs, availability of local guidelines and updated microbiological data, infection control policy, structural resources, educational activity).

10.5 Patients at High Risk of Failure

Patient factors, such as advanced age, comorbidities, physiological status, influence outcomes are essential in addressing treatment outcome. Defining the patient with intra-abdominal sepsis at high risk of failure is difficult: first, it depends on the definition of failure and, second, the high risk may be attributed to the patient's characteristics such as age, comorbidity or the severity of disease at presentation. In general, high-risk IAI is attributed to patient factors or disease factors, represented by high-risk scores, delayed intervention, inability to obtain source control and HA-IAI [36]. While age alone is not decisive for outcome, elderly patients are at higher risk for adverse outcomes, including death, because of frailty associated with advanced age [37]. Frailty can be difficult to measure in the emergency setting.

Disease severity at presentation is associated with risk of failure or poor outcome. The presence of sepsis or septic shock is a negative prognostic factor and defines a disease process that has become systemic. Several disease-specific scores exist. Moreover, pre-admission functional status is important in predicting the risk of failure: nursing home residents have a several-fold increased risk of adverse outcomes, including death [38].

References

1. Sartelli M, Catena F, Abu-Zidan FM, et al. Management of intra-abdominal infections: recommendations by the WSES 2016 consensus conference. World J Emerg Surg. 2017;12:22.
2. Menichetti F, Sganga G. Definition and classification of intra-abdominal infections. J Chemother. 2009;21(Suppl 1):3–4.
3. Seguin P, Fédun Y, Laviolle B, et al. Risk factors for multidrug-resistant bacteria in patients with post-operative peritonitis requiring intensive care. J Antimicrob Chemother. 2010;65(2):342–6.
4. Augustin P, Kermarrec N, Muller-Serieys C, et al. Risk factors for multidrug resistant bacteria and optimization of empirical antibiotic therapy in postoperative peritonitis. Crit Care. 2010;14(1):R20.
5. Solomkin JS, Mazuski JE, Bradley JS, et al. Diagnosis and management of complicated intra-abdominal infection in adults and children: guidelines by the Surgical Infection Society and the Infectious Diseases Society of America. Surg Infect (Larchmt). 2010;11(1):79–109.
6. Das K, Ozdogan M, Karateke F, et al. Comparison of APACHE II, P-POSSUM and SAPS II scoring systems in patients underwent planned laparotomies due to secondary peritonitis. Ann Ital Chir. 2014;85(1):16–21.
7. Vincent JL, Moreno R, Takala J, et al. The SOFA (Sepsis-related Organ Failure Assessment) score to describe organ dysfunction/failure. On behalf of the Working Group on Sepsis-Related Problems of the European Society of Intensive Care Medicine. Intensive Care Med. 1996;22(7):707–10.
8. Kologlu M, Elker D, Altun H, Sayek I. Validation of MPI and PIA II in two different groups of patients with secondary peritonitis. Hepatogastroenterology. 2001;48(37):147–51.
9. Sartelli M, Abu-Zidan FM, Catena F, et al. Global validation of the WSES Sepsis Severity Score for patients with complicated intra-abdominal infections: a prospective multicentre study (WISS study). World J Emerg Surg. 2015;10:61.
10. De Filippo M, Puglisi S, D'Amuri F, et al. CT-guided percutaneous drainage of abdominopelvic collections: a pictorial essay. Radiol Med. 2021;126(12):1561–70.
11. Bufalari A, Giustozzi G, Moggi L. Postoperative intraabdominal abscesses: percutaneous versus surgical treatment. Acta Chir Belg. 1996;96(5):197–200.
12. Ceresoli M, Coccolini F, Montori G, et al. Laparoscopic lavage versus resection in perforated diverticulitis with purulent peritonitis: a meta-analysis of randomized controlled trials. World J Emerg Surg. 2016;11(1):42.
13. Siewert B, Tye G, Kruskal J, et al. Impact of CT-guided drainage in the treatment of diverticular abscesses: size matters. AJR Am J Roentgenol. 2006;186(3):680–6. Erratum in: AJR Am J Roentgenol. 2007;189(3):512.
14. Singh B, May K, Coltart I, et al. The long-term results of percutaneous drainage of diverticular abscess. Ann R Coll Surg Engl. 2008;90(4):297–301.
15. Sallinen V, Akl EA, You JJ, et al. Meta-analysis of antibiotics versus appendicectomy for non-perforated acute appendicitis. Br J Surg. 2016;103(6):656–67.

16. Oliak D, Yamini D, Udani VM, et al. Initial nonoperative management for periappendiceal abscess. Dis Colon Rectum. 2001;44(7):936–41.
17. Brown CV, Abrishami M, Muller M, Velmahos GC. Appendiceal abscess: immediate operation or percutaneous drainage? Am Surg. 2003;69(10):829–32.
18. Sartelli M, Abu-Zidan FM, Ansaloni L, et al. The role of the open abdomen procedure in managing severe abdominal sepsis: WSES position paper. World J Emerg Surg. 2015;10:35.
19. Demetriades D, Salim A. Management of the open abdomen. Surg Clin North Am. 2014;94(1):131–53.
20. Regner JL, Kobayashi L, Coimbra R. Surgical strategies for management of the open abdomen. World J Surg. 2012;36(3):497–510.
21. Swenson BR, Metzger R, Hedrick TL, et al. Choosing antibiotics for intra-abdominal infections: what do we mean by "high risk"? Surg Infect (Larchmt). 2009;10(1):29–39.
22. Vallicelli C, Santandrea G, Sartelli M, et al. Sepsis team organizational model to decrease mortality for intra-abdominal infections: is antibiotic stewardship enough? Antibiotics (Basel). 2022;11(11):1460.
23. Paul M, Shani V, Muchtar E, et al. Systematic review and meta-analysis of the efficacy of appropriate empiric antibiotic therapy for sepsis. Antimicrob Agents Chemother. 2010;54(11):4851–63.
24. Evans L, Rhodes A, Alhazzani W, et al. Surviving sepsis campaign: international guidelines for management of sepsis and septic shock 2021. Intensive Care Med. 2021;47(11):1181–247.
25. Sartelli M, Chichom-Mefire A, Labricciosa FM, et al. The management of intra-abdominal infections from a global perspective: 2017 WSES guidelines for management of intra-abdominal infections. World J Emerg Surg. 2017;12:29. Erratum in: World J Emerg Surg. 2017;12:36.
26. Taccone FS, Laterre PF, Dugernier T, et al. Insufficient β-lactam concentrations in the early phase of severe sepsis and septic shock. Crit Care. 2010;14(4):R126.
27. Plachouras D, Karvanen M, Friberg LE, et al. Population pharmacokinetic analysis of colistin methanesulfonate and colistin after intravenous administration in critically ill patients with infections caused by Gram-negative bacteria. Antimicrob Agents Chemother. 2009;53(8):3430–6.
28. Freeman CD, Nicolau DP, Belliveau PP, Nightingale CH. Once-daily dosing of aminoglycosides: review and recommendations for clinical practice. J Antimicrob Chemother. 1997;39(6):677–86.
29. Klevens RM, Morrison MA, Nadle J, et al. Invasive methicillin-resistant Staphylococcus aureus infections in the United States. JAMA. 2007;298(15):1763–71.
30. Prkno A, Wacker C, Brunkhorst FM, Schlattmann P. Procalcitonin-guided therapy in intensive care unit patients with severe sepsis and septic shock—a systematic review and meta-analysis. Crit Care. 2013;17(6):R291.
31. Knoke M. Gastrointestinale Mikroökologie des Menschen und Candida [Gastrointestinal microecology of humans and Candida]. Mycoses. 1999;42 Suppl 1:30–34.
32. Dupont H, Paugam-Burtz C, Muller-Serieys C, et al. Predictive factors of mortality due to polymicrobial peritonitis with Candida isolation in peritoneal fluid in critically ill patients. Arch Surg. 2002;137(12):1341–6; discussion 1347.
33. Lortholary O, Renaudat C, Sitbon K, et al. Worrisome trends in incidence and mortality of candidemia in intensive care units (Paris area, 2002–2010). Intensive Care Med. 2014;40(9):1303–12.
34. Garey KW, Rege M, Pai MP, et al. Time to initiation of fluconazole therapy impacts mortality in patients with candidemia: a multi-institutional study. Clin Infect Dis. 2006;43(1):25–31.
35. Bassetti M, Righi E, Ansaldi F, et al. A multicenter multinational study of abdominal candidiasis: epidemiology, outcomes and predictors of mortality. Intensive Care Med. 2015;41(9):1601–10.

36. Shirah GR, O'Neill PJ. Intra-abdominal infections. Surg Clin North Am. 2014;94(6):1319–33.
37. Clegg A, Young J, Iliffe S, et al. Frailty in elderly people. Lancet. 2013;381(9868):752–62. Erratum in: Lancet. 2013;382(9901):1328.
38. Finlayson E, Wang L, Landefeld CS, Dudley RA. Major abdominal surgery in nursing home residents: a national study. Ann Surg. 2011;254(6):921–6.

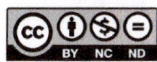

Intra-Abdominal Infections

11

Gabriele Sganga and Christian Eckmann

11.1 Introduction

Intra-abdominal infections (IAIs) represent a common and important cause of morbidity and mortality in the hospital setting, particularly if diagnosed late and/or improperly treated.

In the intensive care unit they are the second most commonly identified site of infection and/or sepsis, preceded by respiratory infections and pneumonia and followed by skin and soft tissue infections.

IAIs account for a wide variety of pathological conditions:

- Infections limited to a single organ (such as cholecystitis, appendicitis, diverticulitis, cholangitis, infected pancreatitis, salpingitis, etc.), which may or may not complicate into peritonitis even in the absence of perforation;
- Peritonitis, based on its extent, is divided into localized or diffuse (generalized);
- Intra-abdominal abscesses, classified based on their location (intraperitoneal, retroperitoneal, parenchymal), anatomical configuration (loculated, multiloculated "walled off") and numerousness (solitary or multiple) [1].

G. Sganga (✉)
Emergency and Trauma Surgery Unit, Fondazione Policlinico Universitario A. Gemelli IRCCS, Università Cattolica del Sacro Cuore, Rome, Italy
e-mail: gabriele.sganga@unicatt.it

C. Eckmann
Department of General, Visceral and Thoracic Surgery, Klinikum Hannoversch-Muenden, Academic Hospital of Goettingen University, Goettingen, Germany
e-mail: chr.eckmann@gmx.de

© The Author(s) 2025
S. Bartoli et al. (eds.), *Infections in Surgery*, Updates in Surgery,
https://doi.org/10.1007/978-3-031-60462-1_11

11.2   Peritonitis

The term "peritonitis" indicates an inflammatory process of the peritoneal meso-thelium, including both chemical (e.g., edematous acute pancreatitis, contamina-tion of the cavity by non-infected gastric juice, etc.) and microbial/infected peritonitis.

The degree of bacterial contamination of the peritoneal cavity depends on the site and cause of the perforation as well as the immune system's ability to contain the infection and the consequent inflammatory cascade. The mesothelium "perito-neum" should therefore be considered an "active immunological organ" capable of reacting to and limiting infection as well as contributing to the exaggerated and uncontrolled cytokine response that leads to septic shock and multiple organ dys-function/failure syndrome.

This is the reason why adequate source control and appropriate antibiotic strat-egy represent the etiological treatments for IAIs which, combined, allow control of the evolution of the septic process.

Peritonitis is generally divided into three categories [1]:

1. Primary peritonitis, also known as spontaneous bacterial peritonitis, is com-monly monomicrobial. It is typical in children where it often mimics appendici-tis (most common causes are pneumococcus and staphylococcus) [2] or in cirrhotic patients with ascites (infected ascites, often due to *E. coli*) or patients on peritoneal dialysis (Tenckhoff catheter infection, often due to *Staphylococcus aureus*), or in tuberculosis or in immunocompromised patients. It is usually associated with moderate mortality and, if recognized, it is treated with antibiot-ics without the need for surgery.
2. Secondary peritonitis is caused by polymicrobial contamination through a perfo-ration, laceration, or necrotic segment of the gastrointestinal tract resulting in bacterial contamination of part or all of the abdominal cavity. The diagnosis is based on history, clinical examination and specific diagnoses can be confirmed by radiographic imaging.
3. Tertiary peritonitis typically occurs in critically ill intensive care or immuno-compromised patients. It represents an infection that is persistent after appro-priate management of primary or secondary peritonitis. It is mostly due to low-grade pathogenic bacteria (enterococci, coagulase-negative staphylococci, *Pseudomonas*, Enterobacterales), fungi (*Candida* species), or low-virulence viruses [1].

11.3   Complicated Intra-Abdominal Infections

When IAI is not promptly recognized and/or treated, its evolution can lead to the body creating inflammatory defense mechanisms, resulting in septic shock and involvement of all organs even distant from the site of infection up to their dysfunc-tion and insufficiency.

The term complicated IAI (c-IAI) is used to indicate secondary infections that, originating from a hollow viscus, extend into the peritoneal space and give rise to an abscess or localized or diffuse peritonitis; their resolution requires both surgical treatment or percutaneous drainage (source control) and systemic antibiotic therapy [1].

Uncomplicated abdominal infections involve intramural inflammation of the gastrointestinal tract without anatomic disruption. However, when treatment is delayed or inappropriate, or the infection involves multidrug-resistant (MDR) bacteria, the risk of progression into a complicated abdominal infection becomes significant.

According to the setting of acquisition and the type of patient and their comorbidities, IAIs can be further divided into:

- Community-acquired c-IAI (CA-IAI): mild-to-moderate and severe forms. It is defined as the development of peritonitis in an outpatient setting. The bacterial flora involved is endogenous and differs based on the organ or site of the gastrointestinal tract involved. The mortality rate of CA-IAI can reach up to 11–29% [3].
- Hospital-acquired c-IAI (HA-IAI): this is defined as an infection that was not present at the time of hospital admission but emerged after at least 48 h in a hospitalized patient, often after surgery, and corresponds to postoperative peritonitis. The mortality rate of HA-IAI and particularly of postoperative nosocomial peritonitis can reach up to 22–55% [3].
- Healthcare-associated c-IAI (HCA-IAIs) [4]: this is defined as an infection present at hospital admission or manifesting within 48 h of admission in a patient with previous contact with healthcare, namely for invasive procedures or dialysis, or who resides in a long-term residential care facility or with a history of MDR infection or colonization, or with an invasive device at the time of admission.

11.4   Microbiology of Complicated Intra-Abdominal Infections

Secondary peritonitis is by definition a polymicrobial infection involving complex microbial communities, consisting of Gram-positive/Gram-negative both aerobic and anaerobic bacteria. Understanding the composition of these microbial communities is essential for guiding empirical antimicrobial therapy and improving treatment outcomes [5, 6].

Moreover, the emergence of MDR organisms has further complicated the management of intra-abdominal infections. MDR organisms, such as extended-spectrum beta-lactamase (ESBL)-producing Enterobacterales and carbapenem-resistant Enterobacterales (CRE), pose a significant threat to patient health and require tailored antimicrobial strategies.

These MDR bacteria are more frequent and typical of hospital-acquired and/or healthcare-associated forms of peritonitis, which is often the case in abdominal sepsis [7]. Moreover, these patient collectives are at risk for invasive abdominal candidiasis [8, 9].

Advancements in diagnostic techniques, such as molecular methods, have facilitated rapid and accurate identification of causative pathogens in intra-abdominal infections. These new microbiological techniques, also known as "fast microbiology", enable clinicians to promptly initiate targeted antimicrobial therapy, thereby improving patient outcomes and reducing the risk of antibiotic resistance.

11.5   Specific Surgical Issues

Early and efficient surgical source control remains the cornerstone of treatment and the most significant prognostic factor in secondary peritonitis [10].

In the context of acute care surgery and the "damage control" approach, procedures such as open abdomen management may be employed to effectively control intra-abdominal septic foci, ischemic bowel, or traumatic injuries. This strategy involves temporarily leaving the abdomen open after initial surgical intervention to address acute conditions like severe trauma or peritonitis.

Open abdomen management allows for continuous monitoring and repeated peritoneal lavage, and it facilitates the management of ongoing inflammation and sepsis. It can prevent or mitigate abdominal compartment syndrome and other complications associated with severe intra-abdominal pathology.

Scheduled relaparotomy, within the framework of damage control surgery, may also be planned to ensure optimal peritoneal cleaning and management of ongoing pathology, thereby improving patient outcomes in cases of severe intra-abdominal sepsis or trauma.

11.6   Conclusions

Early diagnosis and precise identification of the location, extent, and relationships of intra-abdominal sepsis are crucial components of the overall strategy to reduce mortality. Definitive source control through surgical debridement and/or drainage is often the cornerstone of treatment. Timely intervention can prevent the spread of infection, mitigate systemic complications, and improve patient outcomes. In addition to source control, appropriate antibiotic therapy, metabolic and nutritional support, and organ function management, represent a comprehensive and crucially important strategy to promote survival in the management of intra-abdominal sepsis [11].

References

1. Menichetti F, Sganga G. Definition and classification of intra-abdominal infections. J Chemother. 2009;21(Suppl 1):3–4.
2. Cortese F, Fransvea P, Saputelli A, et al. Streptococcus pneumoniae primary peritonitis mimicking acute appendicitis in an immunocompetent patient: a case report and review of the literature. J Med Case Rep. 2019;13(1):126.

3. Mulier S, Penninckx F, Verwaest C, et al. Factors affecting mortality in generalized postoperative peritonitis: multivariate analysis in 96 patients. World J Surg. 2003;27(4):379–84.
4. Klevens RM, Morrison MA, Nadle J, et al. Invasive methicillin-resistant Staphylococcus aureus infections in the United States. JAMA. 2007;298(15):1763–71.
5. Eckmann C, Dryden M, Montravers P, et al. Antimicrobial treatment of "complicated" intra-abdominal infections and the new IDSA guidelines? A commentary and an alternative European approach according to clinical definitions. Eur J Med Res. 2011;16(3):115–26.
6. Eckmann C, Isenmann R, Kujath P, et al. Calculated parenteral initial treatment of bacterial infections: intra-abdominal infections. GMS Infect Dis. 2020;8:Doc13.
7. Blot S, Antonelli M, Arvaniti K, et al. Epidemiology of intra-abdominal infection and sepsis in critically ill patients: "AbSeS", a multinational observational cohort study and ESICM Trials Group Project. Intensive Care Med. 2019;45(12):1703–17.
8. Sganga G, Wang M, Capparella MR, et al. Evaluation of anidulafungin in the treatment of intra-abdominal candidiasis: a pooled analysis of patient-level data from 5 prospective studies. Eur J Clin Microbiol Infect Dis. 2019;38(10):1849–56.
9. Montravers P, Leroy O, Eckmann C. Intra-abdominal candidiasis: it's still a long way to get unquestionable data. Intensive Care Med. 2015;41(9):1682–4.
10. De Pascale G, Antonelli M, Deschepper M, et al. Poor timing and failure of source control are risk factors for mortality in critically ill patients with secondary peritonitis. Intensive Care Med. 2022;48(11):1593–606.
11. Montravers P, Blot S, Dimopoulos G, et al. Therapeutic management of peritonitis: a comprehensive guide for intensivists. Intensive Care Med. 2016;42(8):1234–47.

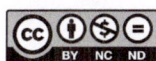

Necrotizing Soft Tissue Infections

12

Francesco Cortese, Stefano Rossi, Maria Cristina Puzzolo,
Caterina Puccioni, Marina Vitillo, Biagio Picardi,
and Simone Rossi Del Monte

12.1 Introduction

Soft tissue infections continue to be a common problem for the healthcare system worldwide, because of their relation with prolonged hospitalization, morbidity and mortality [1]. Necrotizing soft tissue infection (NSTI) can occur in different anatomical locations after a loss of the integrity of the skin (or mucosa) and can be destructive and potentially lethal [2].

Supplementary Information The online version contains supplementary material available at https://doi.org/10.1007/978-3-031-60462-1_12.

F. Cortese (✉) · S. Rossi · C. Puccioni · B. Picardi · S. Rossi Del Monte
Emergency Surgery Unit, San Filippo Neri Hospital, Rome, Italy
e-mail: francescocortese@gmail.com; stefanoro1970@gmail.com;
caterinapuccioni@libero.it; biagiopicardi@gmail.com; rossidelmonte@gmail.com

M. C. Puzzolo · M. Vitillo
Clinical Pathology Unit, San Filippo Neri Hospital, Rome, Italy
e-mail: macripu82@yahoo.it; marina.vitillo@aslroma1.it

12.2 Classification and Epidemiology

Skin and soft tissue infections (SSTIs) are mostly non-complicated infectious processes, such as cellulitis, abscesses or infected wounds. Among them, the complicated forms can be defined NSTIs, described in several classification systems in terms of their anatomic location, causative pathogen(s), rate of progression, depth of infection, and severity of clinical presentation [3, 4]. The WSES guidelines in 2015 proposed a new definition of SSTIs, dividing them into three main groups: surgical site infections (SSIs), non-necrotizing SSTIs, and necrotizing SSTIs (NSTIs) [5]. NSTIs are rare, with an incidence of 4 per 100,000 population per year [6].

Among the NSTIs, it is possible to identify necrotizing cellulitis, necrotizing myositis, and necrotizing fasciitis [1]. Necrotizing cellulitis is usually caused by anaerobic pathogens and can be divided into clostridial and nonclostridial. Necrotizing myositis is an infection of the skeletal muscle usually caused by Group A Streptococcus (GAS). Necrotizing fasciitis is the most common NSTI, with an incidence from 0.3 to 15 cases per 100,000 population according to different studies [7]. Infections can be divided into polymicrobial (type I) and monomicrobial (type II) [8]. Polymicrobial infections are commonly caused by aerobic and anaerobic bacteria, whereas monomicrobial ones are usually caused by GAS or other β-hemolytic streptococci [9]. The extremities are the most frequent region to be involved by necrotizing fasciitis, followed by the perineal region, where it is also known as Fournier's gangrene.

Patients with NSTIs are usually 50–60 years old, with a slight male predominance, and from 4% to 12% of them have a recurrent NSTI [2, 10]. Patients with NSTIs may be critical: up to 50% of them develop septic shock [11]. The mortality rate, which reaches 30% worldwide, is influenced by the virulence of the pathogens and is related to the patient's comorbidities and the affected body region [12, 13].

12.3 Risk Factors

Among the risk factors, it is possible to list [8, 14]:

1. *Weakened immune system*: patients with diabetes, AIDS or cancer are more likely to develop NSTIs.
2. *Recent trauma or surgery*: open wounds provide an entry point for bacteria.
3. *Chronic health conditions, alcoholism.*
4. *Diabetes*: patients affected by diabetes have impaired wound healing and consequently an increased susceptibility to infection. This could be the reason why a critical number of SSTI in diabetic patients present as more serious NSTI (up to 44.5% of patients with NSTI are diabetic).
5. *Injection drug use.*
6. *Age*: both infants and the elderly.

12.4   Causes and Pathophysiology

NSTIs are typically caused by several different types of bacteria, but the most frequently found are *Streptococcus pyogenes* (GAS) and *Staphylococcus aureus*, including methicillin-resistant *S. aureus* (MRSA). Other bacterial pathogens, such as Clostridia and *Vibrio* species, can also cause NSTIs in specific circumstances such as during exposure to warm waters [8].

The potential for the bacteria to cause local tissue injury and a dysregulated systemic inflammatory response is mediated by the release of bacterial toxins, which lead to inflammatory changes in the skin and subcutaneous lymphatics. In the case of necrotizing infections, thrombosis of venules and arterioles causes ischemia and necrosis of the affected tissue [15]. The systemic response to the toxins is characterized by fever from the release of endogenous cytokines and hypotension, which leads to cardiovascular compensatory tachycardia and subsequent inadequate end-organ perfusion. The result is a multi-organ dysfunction in the late phase of the disease [15]. It is this progression of local disease and systemic inflammation that mandates a timely diagnosis and treatment with both appropriate antibiotic agents and surgical debridement [7].

12.5   Microbiology

NSTIs are often categorized according to their causative organisms in [8]:

- Type I infections: polymicrobial infections commonly related to anaerobic, aerobic and facultative anaerobic bacteria acting synergistically.
- Type II infections, usually monomicrobial. *S. pyogenes* (GAS) is the most frequent pathogen found alone in this type of infection, followed by other β-hemolytic streptococci such as *S. dysgalactiae* [16]. When NSTI is related to GAS, almost 50% of the cases are associated with streptococcal toxic shock syndrome (STSS) [17]. In particular, considering this frequent association, the consensus definition of STSS includes also the concept of soft tissue necrosis with necrotizing fasciitis, myositis and gangrene. Some uncommon causes of type II infection are *S. aureus* (including MRSA), Clostridia species., *Vibrio vulnificus*, and other Gram-negative bacilli.

12.6   Clinical Presentation

NSTIs often start with symptoms similar to other skin infections but, differently from those, there is a rapid deterioration of the patient's clinical condition. The clinical presentation varies depending on the location (Table 12.1) and the course (Table 12.2) of the infection [2].

Table 12.1 Clinical pictures of necrotizing skin and soft-tissue infections

Location	Relative frequency[a]	Portal of entry	Main risk factors
Limb (lower > upper)	70%	Trauma Chronic leg ulcer Burns Insect bites Intravenous drug use Blunt trauma Varicella	Age >60 years Male gender Immunosuppression Diabetes Obesity Chronic lower limb ischemia
Perineal/genital (Fournier's gangrene)	15%	Cutaneous Digestive Urinary/genital	Diabetes Obesity
Cervical	<5%	Tonsillar phlegmon Dental abscess Gland infection	Glucocorticoids
Thoraco-abdominal	<5%	Postoperative	Diabetes Obesity
Orbital	<5%		Diabetes Trauma

Reproduced with permission from [2]

[a] The reported figures are estimates and may vary depending on local patient recruitment and case mix

Table 12.2 Signs and symptoms of necrotizing skin and soft-tissue infections, according to the course of the disease

Early	Late	Very late
Fever	Purple discoloration	Frank necrosis
Pain	Hemorrhagic bullae	Dishwasher pus
Erythema/warmth	Crepitus	Hypoesthesia
Tenderness	Hypotension	
Induration	Organ failures	

Reproduced with permission from [2]

Common symptoms include [14, 18]:

1. severe pain out of proportion relative to the examination findings (72% of cases);
2. rapidly spreading red or purple discoloration with erythema (without sharp margins in 72% of cases);
3. edema that extends beyond the visible erythema (75% of cases): marked edema may produce a compartment syndrome;
4. blisters, ulcers, or black spots on the skin (38% of cases). Within three to five days after onset, skin breakdown with bullae (containing thick pink or purple fluid) and frank cutaneous gangrene can be seen;
5. fever, chills, and general malaise (up to 60% of cases);
6. crepitus (in 50% of cases): subcutaneous gas is often present in type I forms of necrotizing fasciitis, particularly in patients with diabetes;
7. nausea, vomiting, and diarrhea.

In addition to all these generic findings, it is possible to detect more typical findings such as the involvement of the epidermis, dermis, subcutaneous tissue, fascia, and

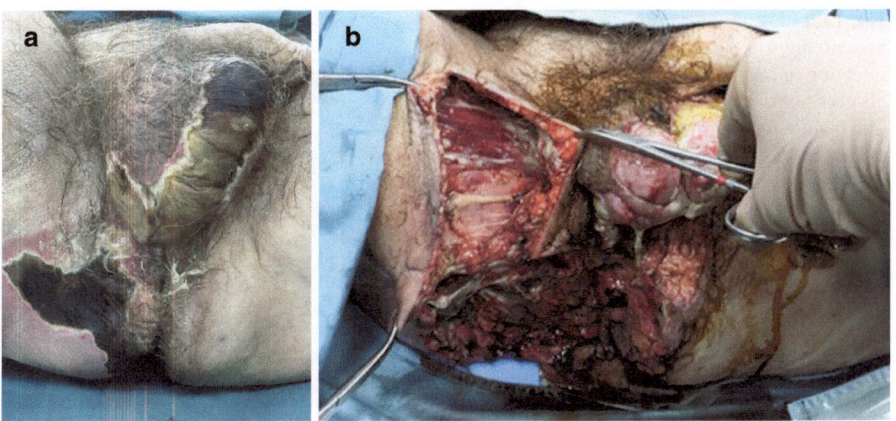

Fig. 12.1 Fournier's gangrene in a diabetic 80-years-old patient. (**a**) Preoperative view of the completely necrotized areas. (**b**) View after source control surgery with complete removed necrotized tissue and no bleeding points

muscle [7]. Necrotizing infection usually presents acutely (over hours) and only rarely it may present subacutely (over days). Prompt progression to extensive destruction can follow, leading to systemic toxicity, limb loss, and/or death [19].

As stated, the most common type of NSTIs is necrotizing fasciitis. Necrotizing fasciitis most frequently involves the extremities. Other presentations include necrotizing fasciitis of the perineum, head and neck region, and neonatal infection.

1. *Perineum* (Fournier's gangrene, Fig. 12.1). This is usually a polymicrobial (type I) form of NSTI. It can occur as a result of a breach in the integrity of the rectal or urethral mucosa that find a communication with the subcutaneous and cutaneous tissue [20]. Fournier's gangrene typically begins suddenly with severe pain and may spread fast to the anterior abdominal wall and the gluteal muscles. Men are more commonly affected than women. In men, the infection usually involves the scrotum and penis; in women it may affect the labia.
2. *Head and neck region.* Necrotizing fasciitis of the head and neck is very uncommon and it can result from a breach in the integrity of the oropharyngeal mucous membrane, usually following surgery or after dental care [21]. Most of the cervical region infections are attributable to mixed aerobic and anaerobic bacteria, although monomicrobial (type II) infection due to GAS can also occur. The majority of reported cases were of dental origin (78%); the remaining cases were of pharyngeal origin or occurred after surgery or trauma [22]. Sometimes fasciitis can spread to the face (according to the study, in up to 22% of cases), lower neck (up to 56%), and mediastinum (up to 40%). Factors that contribute to mediastinal involvement included the use of corticosteroids, infection by gas-producing microbes, and a pharyngeal focus of infection [23]. Other conditions that can arise in the setting of necrotizing infection involving the head and neck region include Ludwig's angina (submandibular space infection) and Lemierre's syndrome (septic thrombophlebitis of the jugular vein).

Fig. 12.2 Escherichia coli necrotizing soft tissue infection in nondiabetic, 50-years-old, male patient. The patient had a polymicrobial infection with *Proteus mirabilis*, *Bacteroides thetaiotaomicron*, *Enterococcus faecium*, and carbapenemase-producing *Acinetobacter baumannii*

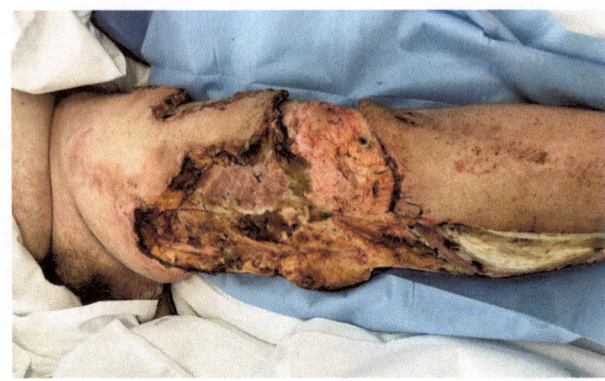

3. *Extremities* (Fig. 12.2). This is the most commonly affected anatomical region (according to the study, up to 57.8% of all necrotizing fasciitis cases) and presentation is usually fulminant. Usually the lower limbs are more involved (68%), but the upper limbs are associated with a higher rate of amputation [24, 25].

12.7 Diagnosis

There are several conditions related to the presentation of NSTIs such as diabetes mellitus, renal failure, arterial occlusive disease, intravenous drug abuse, obesity, liver disease, immunosuppression, recent surgery and traumatic wounds, including minor lesions like insect bites and injection sites [26]. A prompt diagnosis is crucial considering that a delay in diagnosis and consequently in treatment of these infections increases considerably the risk of mortality.

It is crucial to differentiate cellulitis, which can be treated conservatively, from NSTI, which requires immediate operative intervention. The classical clinical presentation described above should be kept in mind, especially the triad of swelling, erythema and disproportionately severe pain, because it can help to raise the suspicion of NSTI [8]. The clinical picture may worsen very quickly, sometimes within hours.

Laboratory tests are not highly sensitive or specific for NSTIs. A rapidly progressive soft tissue infection should be treated as a necrotizing infection from the beginning, because it is better to overestimate it that to underestimate it.

The Laboratory Risk Indicator for Necrotizing infection (LRINEC) score has been proposed to help clinicians in the diagnostic process. The LRINEC score assigns points for abnormalities in six independent variables: serum C-reactive protein level (>150 mg/L), white blood cell (WBC) count (<15,000/μL, 15,000–25,000/μL, >25000/μL), hemoglobin level (≤10.9 g/dL, 11–13.5 g/dL, ≥13.6 g/dL), creatinine level (1.6 mg/dL [142 μmol/L]), sodium level (<135 mmol/L, ≥135 mmol/L), and serum glucose level (>180 mg/dL [10 mmol/L]) [27]. A score of 8 or higher means that the patient has a 75% risk of presenting an NSTI. The real utility of the LRINEC score has been analyzed in several studies. The majority of them have

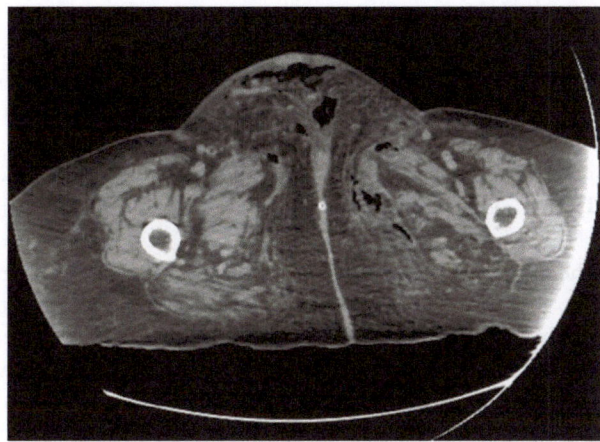

Fig. 12.3 Abdominal TC scan in an obese diabetic 83-years-old patient with chronic atrial fibrillation. Note the pathognomonic air bubbles in the soft tissues of abdominal-pelvic zone and in the left tight

assessed the utility of LRINEC as an additional tool for the early diagnosis of necrotizing infections, considering that a low score does not rule out the diagnosis [28].

For that reason, over the years several studies have tried to identify some other tools that may help in the diagnostic process. Wu et al. investigated the possible role of assaying inflammatory markers in infectious fascia fluid in order to discriminate between cellulitis and necrotizing infections. They found in their limited number of patients that the values of lactate and lactate dehydrogenase (LDH) have a specificity and sensitivity of 100% and 76.9% for lactate and 83.3 and 92.3% for LDH, respectively, in predicting a diagnosis of NSTI [29]. Another marker that is useful in the diagnostic process but even more in evaluating the effectiveness of the debridement and surgical source control, is procalcitonin (PCT). Specifically, the ratio between the preoperative and postoperative PCT values is significantly higher in patients treated successfully, demonstrating that it may considered a clinical tool to evaluate the efficacy of the surgical treatment [30].

In addition to the laboratory findings, radiology has a crucial role during the diagnostic process. Standard X-ray and CT scan help with the diagnosis of NSTIs, by showing gas in 47.9% and 70.3% of cases, respectively (Fig. 12.3) [31, 32]. More specifically, the CT scan has up to 100% sensitivity, 98% specificity, 76% positive predictive value and 100% negative predictive value in identifying NSTI [33]. The diagnostic performance of the CT scan seems to be exceeded by magnetic resonance imaging (MRI) [34]. Ultrasound (US), better if point-of-care US (POCUS), can add useful information to the diagnostic process, in particular by helping in the differential diagnosis between simple cellulitis and NSTIs. This method still has poor accuracy levels as it depends on the experience and skill of the radiologist performing the examination [26]. At the same time, US can assist in the therapeutic process, by guiding the drainage of fluid if detected.

In addition to radiological tools, there are some other more invasive methods, such as fascial biopsy with frozen section and the finger test. The finger test is a surgical diagnostic method, performed at the bedside using local anesthesia. It consists of a 2-cm-long incision deep into the fascia. It is considered positive if there is only minimal or completely absent resistance to finger dissection, with particulate fluid (like "dishwater") and/or necrotic tissue and without bleeding [5].

Although fascial biopsy could add precise information to the diagnostic process, it requires too much time and is not practical in such a time-dependent disease.

12.8   Treatment

The cornerstones of treatment are: prompt surgical source control, adequate antibiotic therapy, and supportive measures with intensive care, if needed [5]. Ideally, surgical source control with proper debridement achieved within 6 h after admission is associated with a mortality rate of 19%, compared with 32% in patients treated later than 6 h [35]. Debridement should be performed in the operating room so as to obtain the best exposure without pain for the patient, achieving complete removal of the necrotic tissue. The skin-sparing debridement techniques seem to be just as effective as the more destructive techniques, but they result in a higher rate of wound closures. Re-explorations should be performed every 12–24 h until the debridement is no longer needed [5]. During the surgical procedure it is crucial to collect deep samples of fascia and necrotized tissues, along with blood cultures, in order to guide the most appropriate antibiotic therapy [2]. When the wound is stable, it is possible to continue the wound care with the aid of negative pressure wound therapy, which reduces the wound surface and promotes granulation.

In conjunction with surgical therapy, it is crucial to start aggressive broad-spectrum empiric antimicrobial therapy, due to the impossibility to define immediately whether it is a type I or type II NSTI [5]. In this light, it is necessary to cover Gram-positive, Gram-negative, and anaerobic organisms until the culture results become available and the antimicrobial therapy can be adjusted.

Despite surgical debridement, antimicrobial therapy, and critical care advancements, NSTI continues to carry a high mortality. Some new treatments have been explored, such as hyperbaric oxygen (HBO) therapy, which appears to be useful despite the lack of published randomized trials. The literature emphasizes that, if available, HBO may be useful provided that it does not delay other available treatments [36]. Intravenous immunoglobulins have also been studied, especially in invasive GAS infections with or without streptococcal toxic shock syndrome [37]. If NSTI is responsible for septic shock, the new guidelines of the Survival Sepsis Campaign should be applied [38]. Patients with NSTI usually need intensive care, with a daily multidisciplinary reassessment of their condition and a multidisciplinary management [39].

References

1. Duane TM, Huston JM, Collom M, et al. Surgical Infection Society 2020 updated guidelines on the management of complicated skin and soft tissue infections. Surg Infect (Larchmt). 2021;22(4):383–99.
2. Peetermans M, de Prost N, Eckmann C, et al. Necrotizing skin and soft-tissue infections in the intensive care unit. Clin Microbiol Infect. 2020;26(1):8–17.

3. Pollack CV Jr, Amin A, Ford WT Jr, et al. Acute bacterial skin and skin structure infections (ABSSSI): practice guidelines for management and care transitions in the emergency department and hospital. J Emerg Med. 2015;48(4):508–19.

4. Eron LJ, Lipsky BA, Low DE, et al. Managing skin and soft tissue infections: expert panel recommendations on key decision points. J Antimicrob Chemother. 2003;52(Suppl 1):i3–i17.

5. Sartelli M, Guirao X, Hardcastle TC, et al. 2018 WSES/SIS-E consensus conference: recommendations for the management of skin and soft-tissue infections. World J Emerg Surg. 2018;13:58.

6. Anaya DA, Dellinger EP. Necrotizing soft-tissue infection: diagnosis and management. Clin Infect Dis. 2007;44(5):705–10.

7. Stevens DL, Bryant AE. Necrotizing soft-tissue infections. N Engl J Med. 2017;377(23):2253–65.

8. Stevens DL, Baddour LM. Necrotizing soft tissue infections. UpToDate. 2022.

9. Stevens DL. Streptococcal toxic-shock syndrome: spectrum of disease, pathogenesis, and new concepts in treatment. Emerg Infect Dis. 1995;1(3):69–78.

10. Endorf FW, Supple KG, Gamelli RL. The evolving characteristics and care of necrotizing soft-tissue infections. Burns. 2005;31(3):269–73.

11. Kao LS, Lew DF, Arab SN, et al. Local variations in the epidemiology, microbiology, and outcome of necrotizing soft-tissue infections: a multicenter study. Am J Surg. 2011;202(2):139–45.

12. Hedetoft M, Madsen MB, Madsen LB, Hyldegaard O. Incidence, comorbidity and mortality in patients with necrotising soft-tissue infections, 2005–2018: a Danish nationwide register-based cohort study. BMJ Open. 2020;10(10):e041302.

13. Nawijn F, Verhiel SHWL, Lunn KN, et al. Factors associated with mortality and amputation caused by necrotizing soft tissue infections of the upper extremity: a retrospective cohort study. World J Surg. 2020;44(3):730–40.

14. Wong CH, Chang HC, Pasupathy S, et al. Necrotizing fasciitis: clinical presentation, microbiology, and determinants of mortality. J Bone Joint Surg Am. 2003;85(8):1454–60.

15. Brook I, Frazier EH. Clinical and microbiological features of necrotizing fasciitis. J Clin Microbiol. 1995;33(9):2382–7.

16. Wall DB, Klein SR, Black S, de Virgilio C. A simple model to help distinguish necrotizing fasciitis from nonnecrotizing soft tissue infection. J Am Coll Surg. 2000;191(3):227–31.

17. Darenberg J, Luca-Harari B, Jasir A, et al. Molecular and clinical characteristics of invasive group A streptococcal infection in Sweden. Clin Infect Dis. 2007;45(4):450–8.

18. Stevens DL, Bisno AL, Chambers HF, et al. Practice guidelines for the diagnosis and management of skin and soft tissue infections: 2014 update by the Infectious Diseases Society of America. Clin Infect Dis. 2014;59(2):147–59.

19. Chelsom J, Halstensen A, Haga T, Høiby EA. Necrotising fasciitis due to group A streptococci in western Norway: incidence and clinical features. Lancet. 1994;344(8930):1111–5.

20. Laucks SS 2nd. Fournier's gangrene. Surg Clin North Am. 1994;74(6):1339–52.

21. Gunaratne DA, Tseros EA, Hasan Z, et al. Cervical necrotizing fasciitis: Systematic review and analysis of 1235 reported cases from the literature. Head Neck. 2018;40(9):2094–102.

22. Mathieu D, Neviere R, Teillon C, et al. Cervical necrotizing fasciitis: clinical manifestations and management. Clin Infect Dis. 1995;21(1):51–6.

23. Petitpas F, Blancal JP, Mateo J, et al. Factors associated with the mediastinal spread of cervical necrotizing fasciitis. Ann Thorac Surg. 2012;93(1):234–8.

24. Nagata K, Shinozaki T, Yamada K, et al. Necrotizing fasciitis of the extremities in high and low Charlson Comorbidity Index: a multi-center retrospective cohort study. J Orthop Sci. 2022;27(5):1056–9.

25. Angoules AG, Kontakis G, Drakoulakis E, et al. Necrotising fasciitis of upper and lower limb: a systematic review. Injury. 2007;38(Suppl 5):S19–26.

26. Goh T, Goh LG, Ang CH, Wong CH. Early diagnosis of necrotizing fasciitis. Br J Surg. 2014;101(1):e119–25.

27. Wong CH, Khin LW, Heng KS, et al. The LRINEC (Laboratory Risk Indicator for Necrotizing Fasciitis) score: a tool for distinguishing necrotizing fasciitis from other soft tissue infections. Crit Care Med. 2004;32(7):1535–41.
28. Fernando SM, Tran A, Cheng W, et al. Necrotizing soft tissue infection: diagnostic accuracy of physical examination, imaging, and LRINEC score: a systematic review and meta-analysis. Ann Surg. 2019;269(1):58–65.
29. Wu KH, Wu PH, Chang CY, et al. Differentiating necrotizing soft tissue infections from cellulitis by soft tissue infectious fluid analysis: a pilot study. World J Emerg Surg. 2022;17(1):1.
30. Friederichs J, Hutter M, Hierholzer C, et al. Procalcitonin ratio as a predictor of successful surgical treatment of severe necrotizing soft tissue infections. Am J Surg. 2013;206(3):368–73.
31. Leichtle SW, Tung L, Khan M, et al. The role of radiologic evaluation in necrotizing soft tissue infections. J Trauma Acute Care Surg. 2016;81(5):921–4.
32. Bruls RJM, Kwee RM. CT in necrotizing soft tissue infection: diagnostic criteria and comparison with LRINEC score. Eur Radiol. 2021;31(11):8536–41.
33. Martinez M, Peponis T, Hage A, et al. The role of computed tomography in the diagnosis of necrotizing soft tissue infections. World J Surg. 2018;42(1):82–7.
34. Kwee RM, Kwee TC. Diagnostic performance of MRI and CT in diagnosing necrotizing soft tissue infection: a systematic review. Skeletal Radiol. 2022;51(4):727–36.
35. Nawijn F, Smeeing DPJ, Houwert RM, et al. Time is of the essence when treating necrotizing soft tissue infections: a systematic review and meta-analysis. World J Emerg Surg. 2020;15:4.
36. Eskes A, Vermeulen H, Lucas C, Ubbink DT. Hyperbaric oxygen therapy for treating acute surgical and traumatic wounds. Cochrane Database Syst Rev. 2013;(12):CD008059.
37. Linnér A, Darenberg J, Sjölin J, et al. Clinical efficacy of polyspecific intravenous immunoglobulin therapy in patients with streptococcal toxic shock syndrome: a comparative observational study. Clin Infect Dis. 2014;59(6):851–7.
38. Evans L, Rhodes A, Alhazzani W, et al. Surviving sepsis campaign: international guidelines for management of sepsis and septic shock 2021. Intensive Care Med. 2021;47(11):1181–247.
39. Urbina T, Madsen MB, de Prost N. Understanding necrotizing soft tissue infections in the intensive care unit. Intensive Care Med. 2020;46(9):1739–42.

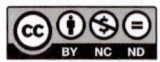

Invasive Candidiasis in Surgery

13

Alessandra Oliva and Mario Venditti

13.1 Introduction

Invasive *Candida* infections (ICIs)—which refer to infections sustained by *Candida* spp. and other fungal species formerly classified as *C. glabrata* (now *Nakaseomyces glabrata*), *C. krusei* (now *Pichia kudriavzevii*), *C. lusitaniae* (now *Clavispora lusitaniae*) and *C. guillermondii* (now *Meyerozyma guilliermondii*)—include three clinical conditions: candidemia only, deep-seated candidiasis, and deep-seated candidiasis with concomitant candidemia [1]. The majority of ICIs are often hospital acquired, especially in critically ill patients [1].

Over recent decades, ICIs have undergone a series of significant epidemiological and clinical changes [1]. On one hand, the population at high risk of ICI, such as immunocompromised and frail patients, those with implants and patients with recent abdominal surgery, has increased; on the other, unlike in the past, the clinical manifestations of ICI have widely diversified, ranging from candidemia only to an array of invasive life-threatening infections possibly involving all body districts [1].

The global incidence of ICIs has shown an overall increase; however, although *Candida albicans* still represents the most common species, an important epidemiological shift towards *non-albicans Candida* species (NAC) has been observed [1]. Despite the recent advancements in diagnosis and treatment, ICIs are still associated with unacceptably high mortality rates and significant increases in healthcare costs [1].

Furthermore, an alarming increase in the rate of resistance to antifungals has been described, involving, above all, *C. parapsilosis* and fluconazole resistance

A. Oliva (✉)
Department of Public Health and Infectious Diseases, Sapienza University of Rome, Rome, Italy
e-mail: alessandra.oliva@uniroma1.it

M. Venditti
Formerly at Department of Public Health and Infectious Diseases, Sapienza University of Rome, Rome, Italy
e-mail: mario.venditti111@gmail.com

© The Author(s) 2025
S. Bartoli et al. (eds.), *Infections in Surgery*, Updates in Surgery,
https://doi.org/10.1007/978-3-031-60462-1_13

(described in up to 30% of isolates), and *C. auris*, which is characterized by a frequent rate of resistance to fluconazole, liposomal amphotericin B (L-AmB), and, to a lesser extent, echinocandins. Multidrug-resistant and pandrug-resistant phenotypes have also been described in *C. auris*. *N. glabrata* shows higher echinocandin resistance than other *Candida* species due to the preferential use of echinocandins for the treatment of these infections, encouraged by increasing azole resistance in this species [1]. Notably, *N. glabrata* possesses a high propensity to mutate *in vivo*, especially in cases of intra-abdominal infections [1].

This chapter reviews the epidemiology and pathogenesis of ICIs in surgery, with special reference to the principal ICIs observed in surgical patients, such as intra-abdominal candidiasis (IAC), prosthetic-valve endocarditis (PVE), prosthetic joint infections (PJIs) and shunt-related meningitis. Central line-related candidemia recognizes specific risk factors in surgical patients, especially with regard to a previous intra-abdominal surgery, which may favor firstly the passage of *Candida* spp. from the gut into the systemic circulation and subsequently, thanks to the ability of *Candida* spp. to produce biofilm, central-line colonization and infection. However, the clinical presentation and treatment of candidemia are not specific for surgical patients but, rather, are similar to those of non-surgical populations. Therefore, in this chapter we did not review candidemia since several other comprehensive reviews on this topic have been published to date [1].

13.2   Epidemiology of Invasive *Candida* Infections in Surgery

The epidemiology of ICIs (with or without concomitant candidemia) is still a difficult and unsolved issue, due to variability in definitions, diagnostic issues and difficulties in differentiating colonization from infection [1]. Furthermore, many cases of ICI may remain underdiagnosed given that only a minority of deep-seated infections are detected by blood cultures.

Most commonly, ICIs are observed in the ICU setting, with a cumulative incidence of 7.07 episodes per 1000 ICU admissions, and, among the patients without concomitant candidemia, approximately 80% suffer from IAC [1]. *C. albicans* was the most frequently isolated species, followed by *N. glabrata* and *C. parapsilosis* [1].

13.3   Pathogenesis of Invasive *Candida* Infections in Surgery

ICIs may present with or without candidemia, and the most common pathogenic mechanisms underlying the development of ICIs in surgical patients may be divided into the exogenous and endogenous pathways, according to the modality of infection development, as summarized in Fig. 13.1 [2, 3].

Likewise, the involved *Candida* species and their specific characteristics (i.e., biofilm production, tissue invasiveness, normal habitat and ability to develop *in vivo* resistance) are different (Table 13.1). Indeed, while the endogenous pathway mostly applies to

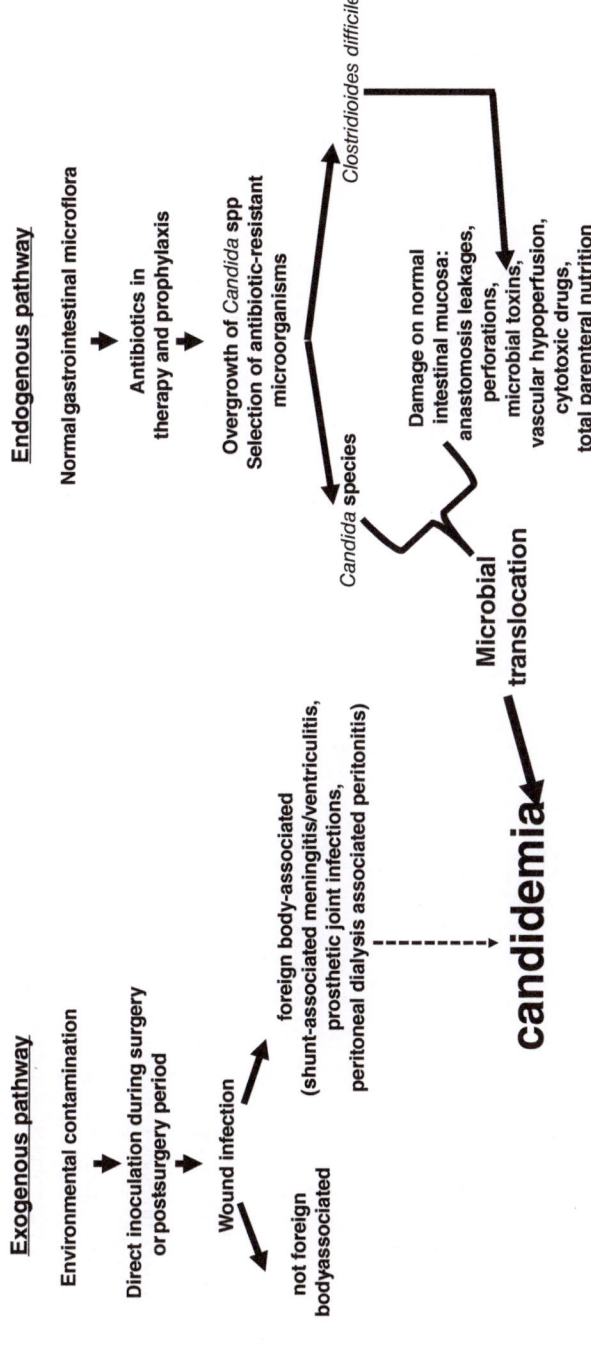

Fig. 13.1 Pathogenic pathways for invasive *Candida* infection with or without candidemia in surgical patients

Table 13.1 Characteristics of *Candida* species involved in invasive disease in surgical patients

Candida species	WHO priority classification [32]	Usual habitat			Exogenous infection	Endogenous infection	Tissue invasiveness	Biofilm production	Isolation trend	Possible antifungal resistance [a]		
		Gastrointestinal tract	Skin	Environment						Fluconazole	Echinocandin	Amphotericin B
Isolated in > 5% of invasive infections												
C. albicans	Critical	+++	+/−	−	+	+++	+++	+++	Decreasing	−	−	−
N. glabrata [b]	High	+++	−	−	+	+++	+++	+++	Increasing	++	++	−
C. parapsilosis complex [c]	High	++	++	+	++	++	++	+++	Increasing	+++	−	−
C. tropicalis	High	+++	+/−	−	+	+++	++++	+++	Stable	++	+	−
Isolated in ≤ 5% of invasive infections												
P. kudriavzevii [b]	Medium	++	−	−	−	++	+	++	Stable	+++	−	−
C. lusitaniae [b]		+	+	++	+	+	++	++	Stable	−	−	+
C. auris	Critical	−	+	++	++	−	+	+++	Emerging	+++/++++	+++	+++
C. haemulonii complex [d]		−	+	++	++	−	+	+++	Emerging	++	+++	+
M. guilliermondii [b] complex [e]		+	−	−	−	+	+	++	Stable	+	+	++

[a] Criteria for resistance scores [3, 33–40]: (1) Fluconazole resistance scores: <1%; + 1–5%; ++ 5–25%; +++ 5–50%; ++++ 90–100%. (2) Echinocandin resistance scores: <0.7; + 0–1.5%; ++ 0–5%; +++ 2–8%. (3) Amphotericin B resistance scores: sporadic; + usually susceptible but resistance may be acquired during therapy; ++ up to 12%; +++ 15–30%

[b] *Nakaseomyces glabrata* (formerly *C. glabrata*); *Pichia kudriavzevii* (formerly *C. krusei*), *Clavispora lusitaniae* (formerly *C. lusitaniae*), *Meyerozyma guilliermondii* (formerly *C. gulliermondii*)

[c] *C. parapsilosis* complex: *C. parapsilosis* sensu stricto, *C. metapsilosis, C. orthopsilosis*

[d] *C. haemulonii* complex: *C. haemulonii* sensu stricto, *C. duobushaemulonii, C. pseudohaemulonii, C. vulturna, C. vulnera, C. khanbhai*

[e] *Meyerozyma guilliermondii* complex: *M. guilliermondii* sensu stricto, *M. carpophila, M. caribbica*

C. albicans, C. tropicalis, N. glabrata and, to a lesser extent, to *C. parapsilosis, P. kudri-avzevii, C. lusitaniae* and *M. guillermondii,* the exogenous pathway is mostly typical of *C. parapsilosis, C. auris, C. haemulonii. Candida* species involved in the exogenous pathway typically share the ability to survive and colonize the environment and/or the skin, potentially causing intra-hospital dissemination and clonal outbreaks [1].

13.4   Specific Types of *Candida* Infections in Surgery

13.4.1 Intra-Abdominal Candidiasis

IAC, which mostly includes peritonitis and intra-abdominal abscesses, accounts for the majority of deep-seated cases of ICI. Approximately 30% of IAC occur in the ICU setting, especially the surgical ones, and only a minority of cases are associated with concomitant candidemia [1]. The most common species is *C. albicans,* followed by *N. glabrata* and, to a lesser extent, *C. tropicalis* and *C. parapsilosis* [1, 4]. IAC is associated with mortality rates around 25–60% [1, 4].

The diagnosis of IAC may be challenging, since clinical signs are not specific and timely microbiological diagnosis is still an issue. A definite diagnosis of IAC requires the isolation of *Candida* spp. from intra-abdominal specimens obtained by percutaneous aspiration or during surgery or the growth of *Candida* from blood cultures in the presence of secondary or tertiary peritonitis in the absence of other pathogens [5]. However, culture may be negative; in these conditions, *Candida* colonization, clinical prediction scores and/or positive non-culture-based diagnostics [i.e., 1–3 β-D-glucan (BDG), T2 Candida, or the combination of the two methods] may help to diagnose IAC [1].

Intestinal perforation, anastomotic leaks, repeated laparotomies, necrotizing pancreatitis and liver/kidney transplants are considered specific risk factors for IAC [4].

A recent retrospective, matched case–control study was conducted in order to identify risk factors associated with IAC in ICU patients. The authors confirmed that concomitant candidemia was observed in only a minority of patients (6.9%), while fluconazole resistance was present in 26.5% of tested isolates [4]. The study confirmed that the risk factors independently associated with IAC were recurrent gastrointestinal perforation, anastomotic leakage and prior use of antifungal drugs or antibiotics, supporting the existing recommendation to consider an antifungal treatment for patients with recent abdominal surgery and recurrent gastrointestinal perforation or anastomotic leakage [4].

An adequate source control and timely adequate antifungal therapy represent the most important drivers of survival [1, 4]. As a general concept, the initial treatment of IAC, especially when presenting acutely, requires intravenous fungicidal drugs such as echinocandins, with or without azoles, or L-AmB [1], while azoles are the preferred step-down agents for maintenance therapy. Similar to echinocandin, L-AmB is a fungicidal agent with high activity against *Candida* species and a low potential for drug-drug interactions, but it is more nephrotoxic than echinocandins.

Therefore, the choice to prefer L-AmB over echinocandins in IAC may be based on its wide tissue penetration in the peritoneal fluid, superior to that of echinocandin, and the consequent lower risk of selecting resistant strains [5]. Indeed, IAC is considered a hidden reservoir for the emergence of echinocandin-resistant *Candida* species, especially in cases of delayed or absent source control, probably as a consequence of prolonged subinhibitory echinocandin concentrations. *FKS* mutant *Candida* isolates were recovered *in vivo* from 24% of IAC patients exposed to echinocandin, and this phenomenon was mostly evident for *N. glabrata*, which, unlike other *Candida species*, present an haploid rather than diploid genome [6]. A recent interesting pre-emptive strategy in patients with suspected abdominal sepsis after abdominal surgery consisted of a loading dose of L-AmB at day 1 (5 mg/kg) followed by normal doses (3 mg/kg) until negative results of BDG or cultures at day 3 [7].

13.4.2 Prosthetic Valve Endocarditis

Candida spp. endocarditis is an uncommon condition that represents <2% of all infective endocarditis, may involve either native or prosthetic valves or intracardiac implantable devices, and often follows a previous candidemia [1, 8]. A recent systematic review including a total of 250 fungal endocarditis, of which 124 (49.6%) were caused by *Candida* species, showed that *C. albicans* and *C. parapsilosis* were the most common (37% and 31.5% of the total, respectively) [8], confirming previous reports on the growing role of *C. parapsilosis* in fungal endocarditis [2]. The authors found that endocarditis on cardiac implants was present in almost half of the cases (45.2%, of which 35.2% on prosthetic valves and 10% on implantable devices) [8]. The mortality rate was 40%, with a relapse rate of 10%.

The clinical presentation of *Candida* endocarditis is not specific and often lacks the signs and symptoms commonly observed in bacterial endocarditis [8]; in addition, *Candida* vegetations are larger and more friable than bacterial ones and are therefore more prone to embolization and metastatic complications [1, 8].

Positive blood cultures along with echocardiography are the diagnostic cornerstone for endocarditis; however, sensitivity of blood cultures may be hampered by previous antifungal therapy and by the longer time needed for a positive result. In these conditions, non-culture methods such as BDG or molecular tests may help in the diagnosis [8].

Giuliano et al. evaluated 140 cases of *Candida* endocarditis, of which 64 (45.7%) were on prosthetic valves. Giving important insights into the pathogenesis of *Candida* endocarditis, the authors found that previous cardiac surgery was associated with PVE, while patients with a history of abdominal surgery and antibiotic exposure were more likely to develop native valve endocarditis (NVE) than PVE. These findings suggested that the first pathogenetic step, common to both PVE and NVE, is *Candida* spp. passage from the gut into the systemic circulation, followed by candidemia, which may be transient and clinically unnoticed, valve colonization and subsequent infection. Therefore, abdominal surgery could be viewed as a factor promoting *Candida* translocation and candidemia for NVE, while in cardiothoracic patients candidemia might be related to translocation following hypoperfusion-related damage of the intestinal mucosa, as occurs during cardiopulmonary bypass and extra-corporeal circulation, especially if longer than 120 min [2].

Interestingly, PVE might be considered a late manifestation of a transient candidemia, possibly occurring several months after surgery. Also, the type of prosthetic valve may have a role in determining the time to endocarditis development, which is longer in mechanical than in biological prostheses, a feature explained by the long time needed for the neoendocardium to form on the mechanical prosthesis [2].

Both *Candida* NVE and PVE are typically a biofilm-associated infection [2]. Interestingly, patients who received moderately and highly active anti-biofilm drugs (L-AmB and echinocandins, respectively) had lower odds of death in endocarditis [2].

Given the high mortality associated with *Candida* endocarditis, a prompt antifungal treatment along with surgery is vital for improving the patients' prognosis. Indeed, Meena et al. demonstrated that combining antifungal treatment with surgery was associated with higher survival rates [8]. Therefore, surgery whenever possible and antifungal treatment with L-AmB or high dose echinocandins, or their combination, followed by oral step-down with fluconazole, is recommended [1]. Chronic suppressive therapy should be considered for patients not eligible for surgery; in these cases, the novel long-acting rezafungin may also have a role [1].

13.4.3 Prosthetic Joint Infections

PJIs are a severe complication of joint surgery involving the prosthesis and contiguous tissues and are associated with high morbidity as they represent the principal reason for joint failure [9]. Fungal PJIs are rare events, occurring in about 1–2% of all cases, with *Candida* spp. being the most common pathogen. However, fungal PJIs are expected to increase owing to the growing rates of prosthetic joint reconstruction, the rise of patients at risk for fungal infections and the increasing use of invasive devices.

While *C. albicans* still represents the most prevalent species, the incidence of NAC causing PJIs has increased over time, in line with other types of ICIs [10]. In particular, a recent systematic review showed that, among the *non-albicans* species, the most frequent was *C. parapsilosis* (54.2%), followed by *N. glabrata* (21.7%) and *C. tropicalis* (12%) [10]. The majority of fungal PJIs are of hematogenous origin while perioperative spread is rarer. The main symptoms of *Candida* PJI are non-specific and often overlap with those of bacterial PJIs. Diagnosis is possible through periprosthetic tissue and/or joint fluid cultures and histopathology,

The surgical and medical approach to fungal PJIs is a real challenge, and no clear guidelines exist. The main indications on the management of these infections come from case series or literature reviews, with a broad range of antifungal and surgical treatments having been reported so far [10]. Currently, the optimal treatment is considered to be the combination of two-stage revision surgery (TSRA) with long-term antifungal treatment [10]. Indeed, TSRA exhibited a higher success rate than the one-stage approach, resection arthroplasty or no surgical treatment [10]. As for antifungals, the majority of infections had been treated with fluconazole, followed by L-AmB and echinocandin. Interestingly, approximately 50% of patients were treated with one antifungal agent, approximately one-third of cases with two agents, either simultaneously or consecutively, and 10% with more than two antifungal agents, with a mean treatment duration of 5.1 months [11]. The drugs of choice for chronic *Candida* PJIs are azoles, while long-acting rezafungin may gain a role for the chronic treatment of these infections in the future [1].

The role of echinocandins in the treatment of *Candida* PJIs was evaluated in a literature review comprising a total of 17 patients treated with echinocandins, 10 as first-choice antifungal therapy and 7 as salvage therapy due to recurrence after initial treatment [9]. The majority of infections were caused by *C. albicans* and *N. glabrata* (7 each), the latter known to be less susceptible to azoles. The duration of echinocandin administration varied considerably (8–90 days, with over half of the patients treated for more than one month). Overall success was observed in all patients, suggesting that echinocandins, thanks to their activity against biofilm [12], may represent an effective and safe treatment for fungal PJIs.

Infection recurrence is a worrying complication of *Candida* PJIs, occurring in 29.6% and 18.3% of patients with hip or knee PJI, respectively [13].

13.4.4 Shunt-Related Meningitis

Meningitis/ventriculitis due to *Candida* spp. is an uncommon but challenging infection, associated with a high mortality rate [14]. Neurosurgical patients are most at risk of *Candida* meningitis/ventriculitis, especially if devices such as external ventricular drains, ventriculoperitoneal shunts or lumbar drains are present [14]. Indeed, the pathogenesis of this condition is based either on hematogenous spread (favored by an altered blood-brain barrier and reduced immunity after neurosurgery) or on colonization of the foreign device during surgery [14].

A recent study, reviewing all cases of meningitis/ventriculitis occurring in a single hospital over a decade, showed that *Candida* spp. was the causative agent of meningitis/ventriculitis in 13 patients. All of these patients had a device *in situ* (external ventricular drain: 11; ventriculoperitoneal shunt: 1; lumbar drain: 1). The most common species was *C. albicans* ($n = 8$), followed by *C. parapsilosis* ($n = 2$), *C. tropicalis* ($n = 1$), and *C. dubliniensis* ($n = 1$), while in one patient culture was negative but 18s rRNA nucleic acid was positive [14].

Being hydrophilic agents, echinocandins have poor penetration across the blood-brain barrier. Consequently, in the presence of *Candida* meningitis/ventriculitis, fluconazole, voriconazole, or L-AmB, either as single agents or in combination, are the preferred therapeutic options [1]. Source control requiring the removal of the infected device is of paramount importance for treatment success.

13.5   Conclusion

The epidemiological and clinical spectra of ICIs have undergone several changes in recent decades, with an increasing rate of NACs as etiological agents and an alarming emerging rate of antifungal resistance. Surgical patients are at risk of specific types of ICI, such as IAC and PVE, which mostly recognize candidemia as the pivotal pathogenetic step, as well as PJI and shunt-related meningitis, which may result from either candidemia or intraoperative contamination as the principal causative pathogenetic steps. Early and appropriate antifungal treatment along with source control are essential for treatment success.

References

1. Oliva A, De Rosa FG, Mikulska M, et al. Invasive Candida infection: epidemiology, clinical and therapeutic aspects of an evolving disease and the role of rezafungin. Expert Rev Anti Infect Ther. 2023;21(9):957–75.
2. Giuliano S, Guastalegname M, Russo A, et al. Candida endocarditis: systematic literature review from 1997 to 2014 and analysis of 29 cases from the Italian Study of Endocarditis. Expert Rev Anti Infect Ther. 2017;15(9):807–18.
3. Oliva A, Aversano L, De Angelis M, et al. Persistent systemic microbial translocation, inflammation, and intestinal damage during Clostridioides difficile infection. Open Forum Infect Dis. 2019;7(1):ofz507.
4. Bassetti M, Vena A, Giacobbe DR, et al. Risk factors for intra-abdominal candidiasis in intensive care units: results from EUCANDICU study. Infect Dis Ther. 2022;11(2):827–40.
5. Felton T, Troke PF, Hope WW. Tissue penetration of antifungal agents. Clin Microbiol Rev. 2014;27(1):68–88.
6. Shields RK, Nguyen MH, Press EG, Clancy CJ. Abdominal candidiasis is a hidden reservoir of echinocandin resistance. Antimicrob Agents Chemother. 2014;58(12):7601–5.
7. Rinaldi M, Bartoletti M, Bonazzetti C, et al. Tolerability of pulsed high-dose L-AmB as pre-emptive therapy in patients at high risk for intra-abdominal candidiasis: a phase 2 study (LAMBDA study). Int J Antimicrob Agents. 2023;62(6):106998.
8. Meena DS, Kumar D, Agarwal M, et al. Clinical features, diagnosis and treatment outcome of fungal endocarditis: a systematic review of reported cases. Mycoses. 2022;65(3):294–302.
9. Lee YR, Kim HJ, Lee EJ, et al. Prosthetic joint infections caused by Candida species: a systematic review and a case series. Mycopathologia. 2019;184(1):23–33.
10. Koutserimpas C, Zervakis SG, Maraki S, et al. Non-albicans Candida prosthetic joint infections: a systematic review of treatment. World J Clin Cases. 2019;7(12):1430–3.
11. Koutserimpas C, Naoum S, Giovanoulis V, et al. Fungal periprosthetic hip joint infections. Diagnostics (Basel). 2022;12(10):2341.
12. Maiolo EM, Oliva A, Furustrand Tafin U, et al. Antifungal activity against planktonic and biofilm Candida albicans in an experimental model of foreign-body infection. J Infect. 2016;72(3):386–92.
13. Gonzalez MR, Bedi ADS, Karczewski D, Lozano-Calderon SA. Treatment and outcomes of fungal prosthetic joint infections: a systematic review of 225 cases. J Arthroplasty. 2023;38(11):2464–71.e1.
14. Kelly L, Walsh J, Skally M, et al. Candida meningitis/ventriculitis over a decade. Increased morbidity and length of stay a concern. Br J Neurosurg. 2023;37(2):227–30.

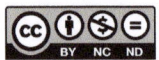

Source Control

14

Silvia Strambi, Camilla Cremonini, Dario Tartaglia,
Massimo Chiarugi, and Federico Coccolini

14.1 Definition

The term "source control" (SC) refers to any intervention aimed at identifying and eliminating (or controlling) the source of infection within the abdomen to restore normal homeostasis [1]. Combined with targeted antibiotic therapy, SC is crucial in the management of intra-abdominal infections (IAIs) [2].

Nowadays, SC is no longer only a surgical concern, but it advocates a multidisciplinary and multimodal approach. A better understanding of sepsis, from its pathophysiological basis to the systemic effects and impact on the human microbiome, implies that SC is a complex concept that encompasses various factors. These include the underlying causative event, the responsible bacteria, the local environment, the overall condition of the patients, and any comorbidities they may have.

The primary objective of SC is to remove or drain the infected material to ensure cessation of the ongoing contamination and further spreading of infection [3]. Moreover, SC aims to manage the production and spread of systemic mediators and the disruptive effects on the microbiome that contribute to multiple organ failure and potentially fatal outcomes.

Despite a good understanding of its complexity, there is currently no conclusive definition of the operative technique, optimal timing, or adequacy of SC, and the morbidity and mortality rates remain high [1].

Supplementary Information The online version contains supplementary material available at https://doi.org/10.1007/978-3-031-60462-1_14.

S. Strambi · C. Cremonini · D. Tartaglia · M. Chiarugi · F. Coccolini (✉)
General, Emergency and Trauma Surgery Department,
Pisa University Hospital, Pisa, Italy
e-mail: silvia.strambi@phd.unipi.it; c.cremonini89@gmail.com;
dario.tartaglia@unipi.it; massimo.chiarugi@unipi.it; federico.coccolini@unipi.it

© The Author(s) 2025
S. Bartoli et al. (eds.), *Infections in Surgery*, Updates in Surgery,
https://doi.org/10.1007/978-3-031-60462-1_14

14.2 Patient Stratification

A proper SC cannot disregard the patient's current physiological condition, medical history, and home therapy. Additionally, the specific source of infection and its clinical severity are dynamic variables that influence the therapeutic strategy. It is therefore evident that SC requires a highly personalized approach. Hence, an initial assessment of the patient based on these variables (physiological condition, comorbidities, medications, immunological status) takes priority.

The WSES Sepsis Severity Score [4] is an easy-to-calculate and specific score for complicated IAIs, which takes into account clinical condition on admission, setting of acquisition, anatomical origin of the IAI, delay in SC and general risk factors (age >70 years, chronic glucocorticoids, immunosuppressant agents, chemotherapy, lymphatic diseases, virus). It represents a useful tool to modulate the extent of SC especially in high-risk patients [4]. The "high-risk" definition is generally used to describe patients with a high probability of treatment failure and mortality.

According to Coccolini et al. [5], patients can more specifically be stratified into three groups:

- *Class A*
- Healthy patients with no or well-controlled comorbidities and no immunocompromise, where the infection is the main problem.
- *Class B*
- Patients with major comorbidities and/or moderate immunocompromise but currently clinically stable, in whom the infection can rapidly worsen the prognosis.
- *Class C*
- Patients with important comorbidities in advanced stages and/or severe immunocompromise, in whom the infection worsens an already severe clinical condition.

In immunocompromised patients, either for congenital or acquired conditions [6, 7] or in the so-called "high-risk patients", it is essential that the evaluation is carried out not only by the surgeon but by a multidisciplinary team, which includes the emergency physician, the anesthesiologist, and the infectious disease specialist, as well as any other specialist consultants depending on the specific pathologies to be evaluated. Once the assessment has been completed, it is the surgeon that has the final responsibility in the decision-making process and who proceeds with SC, if indicated.

14.3 Timing and Priorities

Despite the general agreement to start "as soon as possible", especially in the critically ill patient, to date there is no clear consensus about the timing of SC [1]. Moreover, owing to the need for a tailored approach, general evidence cannot be uniformly applied. There are multiple published indications available, but they lack standardization and the proposed timings for SC vary. It has been proposed that SC should be carried out immediately or "as soon as possible" in patients with severe IAIs, while delayed SC up to 7–24 h after diagnosis has been reported for IAIs without signs of systemic inflammation [2].

The 2017 Surgical Infection Society revised guidelines indicated that SC interventions must be undertaken within 24 h from IAI diagnosis, except when clinical evidence suggests as appropriate a non-interventional or delayed approach (strength of the recommendations: Grade 2-B), whereas a more urgent intervention is warranted in cases of sepsis or septic shock (strength of the recommendations: Grade 2-C) [8]. The guidelines from the Surviving Sepsis Campaign for the Management of Sepsis and Septic Shock recommend promptly determining the anatomical site of infection requiring urgent SC in patients with sepsis or septic shock. They also suggest implementing the necessary SC intervention as soon as it is medically and logistically feasible after the diagnosis is established [1]. The concern previously raised in the literature regarding a possible beneficial effect of delayed treatment in favor of an initial phase of resuscitation and optimization has now been overcome [9–11]. Recent studies on gastrointestinal perforations have confirmed the need for timely treatment, as delays of only 3–6 h were associated with an increase in mortality [1, 12–14]. Boyd-Carson et al. [15] observed that each additional hour of delay of the operative SC caused a 6% increase in mortality and that mortality in patients treated within 6 h was 18% higher than in those treated within the first hour.

The level of urgency of treatment is determined by the site and spread of infection (localized vs. generalized), its rate of progression, and the underlying clinical condition of the patient. Hence, three main situations of SC urgency can be identified [5]:

- *Emergent source control*
- For patients at high risk of mortality due to a severe physiological disturbance caused by the acute disease, emergent SC is necessary and must be initiated as soon as there is strong suspicion or confirmation of the diagnosis.
- *Urgent source control*
- In cases where SC is a critical aspect of infection treatment, it is generally acceptable to delay the intervention for 1–24 h to improve the patient's clinical condition through adequate fluid resuscitation and broad-spectrum antibiotic therapy.
- *Delayed source control*
- SC may be delayed in patients for whom it may be appropriate to wait until the infectious process is clearly delineated, reducing the risks of unintended surgical damage to adjacent tissues.

Any additional SC intervention over the first can be either planned at the time of the initial procedure or decided based on the clinical, laboratory and diagnostic postintervention examinations ("on demand"). Scheduled relaparotomies involve serial surgical revisions every 48–72 h until the abdomen is macroscopically clean, regardless of the patient's clinical status. Their advantages would be the early identification of any residual or recurrent collections and a reduction of the potential risk of gastrointestinal fistulas and delayed hernias. However, this approach comes at the cost of a large number of unnecessary laparotomies [1, 16]. Moreover, additional lavage treatment was demonstrated to have an amplifying effect on the systemic inflammatory mediators (especially IL-8), possibly leading to further organ disfunction [16, 17]. A large 2007 Dutch randomized clinical trial showed positive clinical and economic effects of the on-demand strategy, compared to planned relaparotomy. They observed significantly shorter ICU and median length of hospital stay ($p = 0.001$) combined with a decrease in the rate of relaparotomies and medical costs, with no difference in death or major peritonitis-related morbidity rates [16, 18]. Despite these findings, planned relaparotomies are currently performed. Current evidence suggests the "on demand" strategy as the gold standard in the SC process, based on a careful follow-up with an accurate surveillance algorithm [8].

14.4   Adequacy

There is no universally recognized definition of adequate SC. Adequacy of SC is a broad concept that involves several interrelated requirements, both anatomical and physiological: prompt identification of the site of origin (due to different bacterial flora), gross decontamination (either surgical or not), resolution of the source of infection, proper administration of antibiotics, support of vital functions, and elimination of systemic inflammatory response mediators and toxins [5].

An adequate anatomical and physiological SC must encompass interconnected and combined actions and interventions including [5]:

- antibiotic/anti-infective therapy;
- surgery;
- minimally invasive non-surgical/radiological procedures;
- physiological support and restoration aiming to reduce the disease burden.

Although the treatment varies according to the specific underlying pathology and the patient's clinical condition, a surgical SC associated with short-course antibiotic therapy can be considered sufficient in uncomplicated forms. Otherwise, it could be necessary to extend the duration of antibiotic treatment and physiological support strategies based on the clinical evolution. In severe forms of IAI or in critically ill patients the surgical strategy may involve multiple repeated procedures, until resolution of the infection [5]. In this sense, it may be useful to employ a damage control surgery strategy that provides for the temporary closure of the abdomen associated, if feasible, with a negative pressure wound therapy (NPWT) device [1]. This is particularly indicated to avoid the risk of abdominal compartmental syndrome (ACS) in the presence of intra-abdominal hypertension, to complete SC in persistent infection and to reassess intestinal perfusion in doubtful cases of mesenteric ischemia [8]. Other authors instead underline the risks of leaving open an abdomen which could theoretically be closed, as they argue that ACS in the case of non-traumatic sepsis can be prevented by optimizing medical therapy and that open abdomen increases the risk of fluid and electrolyte imbalances and gastrointestinal fistula [1].

To understand if the open abdomen with NPWT could play a role in improving the clearance of inflammatory mediators in patients, we have to await the results of prospectively randomized trials, such as the COOL Trial [19, 20]. Moreover, the adequacy of SC is also related to the treatment setting, the technologies available in the hospital and the surgeon's skills [2, 5].

14.5 Specific Intra-Abdominal Infections

Figures showing the operative procedures and need for antibiotic therapy based on the patient's classification and urgency level of SC for the main significant sources of IAI (acute cholecystitis, acute cholangitis, acute appendicitis, acute left colonic diverticulitis, acute right colonic diverticulitis, small bowel perforation, gastroduodenal ulcer perforation, post-traumatic perforation, and acute pancreatitis) [5] are provided in the online Supplementary material of this chapter.

References

1. Sartelli M, Coccolini F, Kluger Y, et al. WSES/GAIS/SIS-E/WSIS/AAST global clinical pathways for patients with intra-abdominal infections. World J Emerg Surg. 2021;16(1):49.
2. Schena CA, de'Angelis GL, Carra MC, et al. Antimicrobial challenge in acute care surgery. Antibiotics (Basel). 2022;11(10):1315.
3. Marshall JC, al Naqbi A. Principles of source control in the management of sepsis. Crit Care Clin. 2009;25(4):753–68, viii–ix.
4. Sartelli M, Abu-Zidan FM, Catena F, et al. Global validation of the WSES Sepsis Severity Score for patients with complicated intra-abdominal infections: a prospective multicentre study (WISS study). World J Emerg Surg. 2015;10:61.
5. Coccolini F, Sartelli M, Sawyer R, et al. Source control in emergency general surgery: WSES, GAIS, SIS-E, SIS-A guidelines. World J Emerg Surg. 2023;18(1):41.
6. Coccolini F, Improta M, Sartelli M, et al. Acute abdomen in the immunocompromised patient: WSES, SIS-E, WSIS, AAST, and GAIS guidelines. World J Emerg Surg. 2021;16(1):40.
7. Coccolini F, Improta M, Cicuttin E, et al. Surgical site infection prevention and management in immunocompromised patients: a systematic review of the literature. World J Emerg Surg. 2021;16(1):33.
8. Mazuski JE, Tessier JM, May AK, et al. The Surgical Infection Society revised guidelines on the management of intra-abdominal infection. Surg Infect (Larchmt). 2017;18(1):1–76.
9. Sethi A, Debbarma M, Narang N, et al. Impact of targeted preoperative optimization on clinical outcome in emergency abdominal surgeries: a prospective randomized trial. Anesth Essays Res. 2018;12(1):149–54.
10. Coccolini F, Sartelli M, Catena F, et al. Early goal-directed treatment versus standard care in management of early septic shock: meta-analysis of randomized trials. J Trauma Acute Care Surg. 2016;81(5):971–8.
11. Azuhata T, Kinoshita K, Kawano D, et al. Time from admission to initiation of surgery for source control is a critical determinant of survival in patients with gastrointestinal perforation with associated septic shock. Crit Care. 2014;18(3):R87.
12. Bloos F, Thomas-Rüddel D, Rüddel H, et al. Impact of compliance with infection management guidelines on outcome in patients with severe sepsis: a prospective observational multi-center study. Crit Care. 2014;18(2):R42.
13. De Waele JJ. Early source control in sepsis. Langenbecks Arch Surg. 2010;395(5):489–94.

14. Hecker A, Schneck E, Röhrig R, et al. The impact of early surgical intervention in free intestinal perforation: a time-to-intervention pilot study. World J Emerg Surg. 2015;10:54.
15. Boyd-Carson H, Doleman B, Cromwell D, et al. Delay in source control in perforated peptic ulcer leads to 6% increased risk of death per hour: a nationwide cohort study. World J Surg. 2020;44(3):869–75.
16. van Ruler O, Boermeester MA. Surgical treatment of secondary peritonitis: a continuing problem. Chirurg. 2017;88(Suppl 1):1–6.
17. Zügel N, Siebeck M, Geissler B, et al. Circulating mediators and organ function in patients undergoing planned relaparotomy vs conventional surgical therapy in severe secondary peritonitis. Arch Surg. 2002;137(5):590–9.
18. van Ruler O, Mahler CW, Boer KR, et al. Comparison of on-demand vs planned relaparotomy strategy in patients with severe peritonitis: a randomized trial. JAMA. 2007;298(8):865–72.
19. Kirkpatrick AW, Coccolini F, Ansaloni L, et al. Closed or open after source control laparotomy for severe complicated intra-abdominal sepsis (the COOL trial): study protocol for a randomized controlled trial. World J Emerg Surg. 2018;13:26.
20. Kirkpatrick AW, Coccolini F, Tolonen M, et al. The unrestricted global effort to complete the COOL trial. World J Emerg Surg. 2023;18(1):33.

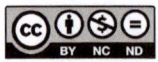

Infection Control in Prosthetic Surgery

15

Giulia Ianni, Francesco Pizza, Andrea Siani,
Tommaso Castrucci, Federico Accrocca,
and Stefano Bartoli

15.1 Introduction

Surgical site infections (SSI) occur in all surgical specialties with an incidence of 2–5% for class 1–2 clean procedures, and account for approximately 38% of all nosocomial infections related to surgery. Higher rates are reported in traumatic injuries (20–50%), in specific conditions, or in patients undergoing high-risk vascular surgery (15% or higher). SSI significantly increase both costs and morbidity, especially when prosthetic material is used [1]. Indeed, in the last two decades, although the advent of endovascular procedures in selected cases would seem to have improved outcomes, graft infection still remains one of the most important adverse events (0.5–5%) and a serious health problem [2]. Mesh infections in ventral hernia repair result in reoperations in 5–10% of cases, leading to longer hospital stays and higher healthcare costs [3].

15.2 Pathogenesis

The pathobiology of SSI is best understood if it is classified as an infection mediated by pathogenic strains that grow and develop by creating a barrier called a "biofilm" [4]. The matrix constituting the biofilm is composed of extracellular polymeric substance (EPS) produced by bacteria and their degradation in contact with the host organism. The bacteria adhere to the prosthetic material forming microcolonies in

G. Ianni (✉) · A. Siani · T. Castrucci · F. Accrocca · S. Bartoli
Department of Vascular Surgery, Sant'Eugenio Hospital-ASL Roma 2, Rome, Italy
e-mail: giuliaianni@hotmail.com; andreasiani@yahoo.it; tcastrucci@gmail.com;
federico.accrocca@aslroma2.it; steba08@gmail.com

F. Pizza
A. Rizzoli Hospital, ASL Napoli 2 Nord, Naples, Italy
e-mail: francesco_pizza@libero.it

© The Author(s) 2025
S. Bartoli et al. (eds.), *Infections in Surgery*, Updates in Surgery,
https://doi.org/10.1007/978-3-031-60462-1_15

which the production of EPS begins; this represents a stable and safe environment in which they live and communicate with each other (quorum sensing mechanism). In this matrix, the bacteria show a low level of both activity and growth, and this explains their high resistance to the host defenses and low sensitivity to antibiotics [4, 5]. The bacterial biofilm is able to colonize potentially all prosthetic surfaces such as heart valves, vascular and orthopedic prostheses and intravenous catheters. According to the National Institutes of Health, it is estimated that 65% of soft tissue, respiratory and urinary tract infections are caused in part by biofilm-producing bacteria [5]. Bacterial adhesion to the prosthetic device is promoted by the fluid proteins present in both the blood and tissues of the host organism, by the characteristics of the prosthetic surface and by the intrinsic properties of the bacterium; in *Staphylococcus* spp., for example, the adhesion process is controlled by specific genes which code for extracellular adhesion proteins. Biofilm formation can occur either by direct contamination or by transient bacteremia. The biofilm formation process involves four stages: (1) adhesion; (2) aggregation and accumulation of EPS; (3) maturation; and (4) detachment.

During the last stage (planktonic phase), the bacteria start to form a new biofilm on a distant surface within the host, thus spreading the infection. The most important aspect that characterizes biofilm is resistance to antibiotic agents. Indeed, antimicrobial agents have greater difficulty penetrating the biofilm because of both the action of the mechanical barrier and the reduced metabolic activity of the bacteria. Some substances such as lactoferrin (chelating iron), N-acetyl cysteine, silver and some antibiotics (rifampicin, macrolides, azithromycin) are able to interfere with the production of biofilms by preventing the nutrition of the bacteria themselves and inhibiting the production of the EPS and communication between cells (quorum sensing inhibitor) [6].

Several studies have been carried out to evaluate the biocompatibility and resistance to infections of prostheses used vascular surgery. Polyethylene terephthalate (Dacron) and polytetrafluoroethylene (PTFE), known as Gore-Tex, are the most commonly used synthetic grafts in vascular surgery. Dacron prostheses have two different textures (woven and knitted) that lead to different permeability, compliance and tissue integration, exposing to a greater risk of infection. The PTFE molecule is biologically stable and, due its electronegative surface, the interaction of blood cells with the prosthesis is minimal, making it more resistant to germs [7]. Many tools have been investigated to prevent or solve the infection, such as the use of antibiotic beads. Initially used to combat possible infections associated with emergency orthopedic surgery and in osteomyelitis, they were subsequently used in prosthetic infections in the vascular field.

Even in abdominal wall surgery the choice of prosthetic materials can make a significant difference.

Synthetic meshes—e.g., made of heavyweight polypropylene (PP), PTFE, combinations of PTFE/PP, PP covered with omega-3 fatty acids (C-QUR mesh), and multifilament polyester—facilitate the formation of biofilm leading to both acute and chronic recurrent infections requiring removal of the mesh. Biological or biosynthetic meshes, although more expensive, have been associated with lower rates of mesh infection, between 1.5% and 10.9% [8].

Unlike powders, pastes and sponges, antibiotic beads have greater stability over time and therefore the release of antibiotic molecules is more lasting. At first, a sort of bone cement (polymethylmethacrylate, PMMA) was used, which was mixed with antibiotic powder and shaped in non-absorbable beads and then either left indefinitely or removed in a later surgical procedure. Subsequently, biodegradable formulations based on calcium sulphate ($CaSO_4$) were used, formulations which dissolve after months, releasing a high antibiotic concentration [1]. With the use of antimicrobial prostheses, the infection will only occur if the bacteria that approach the prosthetic surface are able to adhere to it and become metabolically active. By far the most frequently used are silver prostheses. The antimicrobial efficacy of silver is attributed to a series of mechanisms including the binding to membrane phospholipids which interferes with membrane transport and effectively closes the cell pump mechanism necessary for bacterial cell viability [9].

15.3   Bacteriology

Although any microorganism could potentially be responsible for a prosthetic infection, *Staphylococcus aureus* is involved in approximately 80% of cases of vascular graft, orthopedic or cardiac prosthesis infection, with an approximately four-fold increase in recent decades of methicillin-resistant *S. aureus* (MRSA). Infection can be caused by both Gram-positive and Gram-negative strains; the most frequently found germs are Staphylococci (*S. aureus* and *S. epidermidis*), Streptococci, Enterococci, *Escherichia coli*, *Klebsiella pneumoniae*, Enterobacterales, *Pseudomonas* spp., and *Candida albicans* [10]. Staphylococci and *Pseudomonas* spp. are strong biofilm producers. *S. aureus,* in particular, is a microorganism capable of surviving in highly unfavorable conditions by colonizing the mucous membranes (e.g., the nasal mucosae) and the skin, causing serious pyogenic infections and worse SSI outcomes [11].

15.4   Classification

Depending on the onset, prosthetic infections are classified into early and late. Early infections develop within 3 months from surgery, and manifest with fever, bacteremia, pain, bleeding, erythema and purulent secretion from the surgical site and, in vascular surgery, with graft occlusion or formation of pseudoaneurysms. They are generally due to virulent microorganisms such as *S. aureus*, *E. coli*, *Klebsiella* spp., *Pseudomonas* spp. or other Gram-negative species that spread rapidly and can cause tissue necrosis and rupture of the anastomosis. Late infections develop several months after surgery and can result from a local infection involving the prosthesis or from bacteremia; they generally have milder symptoms, few systemic manifestations and often negative blood cultures. The most frequently encountered bacterium is *S. epidermidis* [12, 13].

Infections starting from the digestive system are generally polymicrobial, involving Gram-positive bacilli and enterobacteria such as *E. coli*, *Klebsiella* spp., *Proteus mirabilis* and *Candida* spp. [10].

Aortic graft infections are rare (1–3%) but associated with a high mortality rate (20–30%); infrainguinal bypasses present a higher percentage of SSI and graft infection (4%) with mortality and amputation rates of 17% and 40%, respectively. Infections secondary to hip or knee replacements occur in 0.3–2.5% of cases [12].

According to Kao et al., the clinical manifestations of mesh infection in hernia surgery can occur either a few days after its implantation or several months or years later, with a prodromal period around 20 months [8].

15.5 Diagnosis

The diagnostic tools most commonly used to diagnose infection of a prosthetic implant include ultrasound, computed tomography (CT) angiography or scintigraphy with labeled leukocytes. Currently, ^{18}F-fluorodeoxyglucose positron emission tomography (FDG-PET) combined with CT imaging (FDG-PET/CT) would seem to be preferable to labeled leukocyte scintigraphy owing to its better specificity and sensitivity [14, 15].

However, CT remains the diagnostic test of choice. CT scans show ectopic gas (considered normal within 6 weeks of surgery), periprosthetic fluid, presence of pseudoaneurysms, thickening of fat and soft tissue (>5 mm) between the graft and the surrounding aneurysm wall. In acute prosthetic infections, the sensitivity of CT is nearly 100%; however, in the case of low-grade prosthetic infections, the risk of false negative results is high. CT-guided puncture can collect periprosthetic fluid for culture and establish a microbiological diagnosis [12].

Magnetic resonance imaging (MRI) was not superior to CT for early infections; there are few comparative studies and these have been done on small patient groups. The difficulties related to this examination are its scarce use in emergency and postoperative settings due to the difficulty differentiating a postoperative hematoma from an early infection [16].

The presence of swelling and chronic pain needs to be evaluated with ultrasound or CT scan. CT scans frequently reveal signs of infection, such as wrinkling or folding of the mesh.

A chronic sinus tract or the visible protrusion of the mesh through the skin are definite signs of a chronic infection [17].

15.6 Infection Control

The 2017 Centers for Disease Control and Prevention (CDC) guidelines for SSI prevention were strictly based on a systematic review of the medical literature evaluated using a modified GRADE (Grading of recommendations, assessment, development and evaluation) in accordance with the 2009 CDC recommendations. The revised and published recommendations in 2017 are classified into five categories based on the level of supporting evidence: strong recommendation (categories IA, IB, and IC); weak recommendation (category II); no recommendations/unresolved [17–19].

The recommendations are categorized into *essential practices* that should be adopted by all emergency care hospitals and *adjunctive practices* when SSIs are not controlled after implementation of essential practices.

The most important recommendations in prosthetic surgery are the following [17, 20, 21]:

- Have the patient take a shower with antiseptic-based soap (chlorhexidine) the evening before the surgical procedure.
- The administration of a correct and effective antibiotic prophylaxis without administering further therapy at the end of the operation for clean and clean-contaminated procedures even in the presence of drainage.
- In the operating setting, careful observation of hand hygiene, use of gloves and other protection devices (masks, gowns and shoes covers) by all operating room personnel is mandatory.
- Patients with evidence of active infection prior to elective surgical procedures should complete treatment for infection prior to surgery, particularly when prosthetic material implantation is planned.
- Although there are no strong indications for screening and decolonization of *S. aureus* with mupirocin ointment applied 3–5 days in advance, this may be reasonable for surgical patients known to be nasal carriers of *S. aureus* or for patients undergoing prosthetic surgery at high risk for adverse outcomes in case of *S. aureus* infection at the surgical site (e.g., cardiothoracic surgery, vascular surgery, orthopedic procedures, immunocompromised patients).
- Wound covers reduce the risk of abdominal SSI and are important for the prevention of SSI during clean, contaminated and dirty abdominal procedures. Minimally invasive/laparoscopic procedures are generally associated with lower SSI rates than open surgery.
- There is insufficient evidence for the routine use of preoperative hair removal or laminar airflow to reduce the risk of SSI.
- Use alcohol-containing preoperative disinfecting agents in combination with an antiseptic to reduce the load on the skin flora.
- There is evidence that regulation of host defense factors—maintenance of normothermia, tissue oxygenation and glucose homeostasis—are important in determining the risk of SSI in an individual patient.
- Do not give transfusions unless necessary to reduce the SSI rate.

Risk factors for developing SSI are divided into preoperative (patient-related), perioperative (procedure-related) and postoperative categories. Patient-related risk factors are modifiable (e.g., poorly controlled diabetes mellitus, obesity, malnutrition, smoking habits, length of preoperative hospitalization, and nasal colonization with *S. aureus*) or non-modifiable (e.g., age). Procedure-related risk factors include wound class (clean, clean-contaminated, contaminated, dirty, infected), organ site and duration of the operation. Postoperative concerns include wound care, postoperative blood transfusions, hyperglycemia in both diabetic and nondiabetic patients and oxygenation status [17]. Obesity, malnutrition and obesity combined with malnutrition increase the risk of infections especially in orthopedic and hernia surgery. Malnutrition is associated with impaired wound healing and immunity, and consequently with an increased risk of infection. An albumin level below 3.5 g/dL, leukocytes below 1500 cells/mm^3, and transferrin levels below 200 mg/dL are widely considered serum markers of malnutrition and should be evaluated and optimized in the preoperative setting. Diabetes mellitus and pre- and postoperative hyperglycemia were more common in patients who develop prosthetic joint infection; postoperative blood glucose levels above 200 mg/dL lead to a two-fold increased risk of infection. Patients with an uncontrolled diabetes mellitus are at higher risk. In addition, preoperative increased levels of glycated hemoglobin and fasting hyperglycemia have been associated with the development of postoperative hyperglycemia. A perioperative blood glucose level of 80 to 180 mg/dL is currently recommended. Smoking significantly increases the risk of prosthetic joint infection, probably as a result of vasoconstriction in the surgical area with impaired wound healing. Abstaining from smoking for more than 4 weeks is strongly recommended. Pre-existing anemia increases the risk of prosthetic joint infection, but it has not yet been shown that preoperative correction will reduce its rate. Preoperative correction of anemia with iron and erythropoietin seems to be a valid alternative to reduce the need for transfusions and consequently the risk of infection [22–24].

15.7   Therapy in Vascular Surgery

Infections involving vascular prosthetic grafts may be superficial if localized at the skin level, deep if involving the subcutaneous tissue, muscle fascia and the graft itself (if located in the groin), or organ/space when a graft is placed deep as in the case of thoracic and abdominal grafts.

Infections are classified as SSIs if occurring within 30 days from a surgical procedure when no graft material is used and if occurring within 1 year when a surgical or endovascular graft is implanted. Two classifications are commonly used in the description of prosthetic vascular infections: Szilagyi's and Samson's. The latter differentiates the involvement of part or all of the graft and the presence or absence of systemic signs of sepsis or bleeding as the first clinical manifestation [22, 25]. The first effort in the presence of SSI is the debridement of the surgical site (source control) and, where possible, the replacement of the infected prosthetic graft. The replacement takes place as first choice, with autologous venous material, with cryopreserved arterial material, with silver-plated or antibiotic-impregnated grafts, as described in numerous, also experimental, studies [9, 25–27]. Although the treatment of choice is the removal and replacement of the infected graft, in some patients with severe comorbidities or where the existing aortic graft is in an anatomical location that precludes excision without causing a high likelihood of morbidity and/or mortality (aortic arch or thoracoabdominal aorta), or in the case of infections mediated by less virulent germs or as a bridging treatment in view of definitive surgery, an alternative conservative approach can be considered as treatment of the infected graft. Some authors have presented excellent long-term results in terms of limb salvage and mortality even in patients undergoing orthopedic surgery, using antibiotic beads to be applied to the surgical site or wound irrigation with antibiotics and antiseptics [28–30]. According to a strong recommendation (category I B) of the guidelines of European Society for Vascular Surgery, antimicrobial therapy should be mandatory in vascular graft/endograft infection [31]. First, antimicrobial therapy with broad spectrum antibiotics is indicated to control infection and sepsis. Once the microorganism responsible for the infection has been isolated, switching to specific antimicrobial therapy should be considered. The fact that the microbial pathogens involved are often biofilm producers must be taken into account when choosing the most appropriate antibiotics. Sometimes the addition of antifungal agents should be considered, especially in cases of visceral fistula [31].

Contraindications to a conservative approach are infected anastomotic aneurysms, aortoenteric fistulas, hemorrhage from suture disruption, or when the infection is due to invasive Gram-negative organisms like *Pseudomonas* spp. or *Salmonella* spp., as the failure rate reaches 75% in these cases [28, 32].

15.8 Therapy in Hernia Surgery

The management of mesh infections in hernia surgery depends on the severity of the infection and the patient's condition. Treatment options may include:

1. *Antibiotic therapy and mesh saving*: percutaneous drainage of fluid collections combined with intravenous administration of antibiotics, local debridement with saline or antibiotic irrigation and the use of vacuum-assisted closure systems (VAC) are possible conservative treatments with acceptable short-term results. The management of heavyweight PP, PTFE, and polyester meshes is more demanding [33].
2. *Mesh removal*: if the infection is chronic and the patient is serious or unstable and does not respond to antibiotic therapy, complete removal of the infected mesh may be necessary. *S. aureus* was detected in 89% of mesh infections (49% MRSA). MRSA infections are difficult to eliminate and are associated with a 2.5-fold reduction in the chance of successful mesh salvage.
3. *Two-stage procedure*: this approach consists of two phases: the first stage involves debridement of the wound, removal of the meshes and antibiotic therapy, while the second stage involves definitive reconstruction of the abdominal wall. Subsequently, a new mesh can be considered in a second procedure (planned ventral hernia). Often the second operation does not take place due the patient's fear, leading to an increase in emergency surgery for complications such as obstruction and fistula [34].

4. *One-stage procedure*: considered dangerous and complex due to the high risk of reinfection even if not universally accepted. The distinction between the types of materials is important: synthetic mesh, organic mesh and bioresorbable mesh. Biological meshes are associated with significant SSI occurrence rates (up to 66%) and by high long-term hernia recurrence rates (50%) [35]. Developed as a potentially cost-effective alternative to synthetic and tissue-derived products, biosynthetic resorbable mesh is particularly useful in cases with a high risk of complex mesh infections. Benefits include a single operation, but there is a risk of re-infection of the meshes [36].

References

1. McGuinness B, Ali KP, Phillips S, Stacey M. A scoping review on the use of antibiotic-impregnated beads and applications to vascular surgery. Vasc Endovasc Surg. 2020;54(2):147–61.
2. Maeda K, Kanaoka Y, Ohki T, et al. Better clinical practice could overcome patient-related risk factors of vascular surgical site infections. J Endovasc Ther. 2015;22(4):640–6.
3. Kokotovic D, Bisgaard T, Helgstrand F. Long-term recurrence and complications associated with elective incisional hernia repair. JAMA. 2016;316(15):1575–82.
4. Bergamini TM. Pathobiology of the graft surface bacterial biofilm. In: Bunt TJ, editor. Vascular graft infection. Armonk: Futura Publishing; 1994.
5. Frei E, Hodgkiss-Harlow K, Rossi PJ, et al. Microbial pathogenesis of bacterial biofilms: a causative factor of vascular surgical site infection. Vasc Endovasc Surg. 2011;45(8):688–96.
6. Welliver RC Jr, Hanerhoff BL, Henry GD, Köhler TS. Significance of biofilm for the prosthetic surgeon. Curr Urol Rep. 2014;15(6):411.
7. Russu E, Mureşan AV, Ivănescu AD, et al. Polytetrafluorethylene (PTFE) vs. polyester (Dacron) grafts in critical limb ischemia salvage. Int J Environ Res Public Health. 2023;20(2):1235.
8. Kao AM, Arnold MR, Augenstein VA, Heniford BT. Prevention and treatment strategies for mesh infection in abdominal wall reconstruction. Plast Reconstr Surg. 2018;142(3 Suppl):149S–55S.
9. Ricco JB, Assadian O. Antimicrobial silver grafts for prevention and treatment of vascular graft infection. Semin Vasc Surg. 2011;24(4):234–41.
10. Hodgkiss-Harlow KD, Bandyk DF. Antibiotic therapy of aortic graft infection: treatment and prevention recommendations. Semin Vasc Surg. 2011;24(4):191–8.
11. Costa Almeida CE, Reis L, Carvalho L, Costa Almeida CM. Collagen implant with gentamicin sulphate reduces surgical site infection in vascular surgery: a prospective cohort study. Int J Surg. 2014;12(10):1100–4.
12. Hasse B, Husmann L, Zinkernagel A, et al. Vascular graft infections. Swiss Med Wkly. 2013;143:w13754.
13. Aboshady I, Raad I, Vela D, et al. Prevention of perioperative vascular prosthetic infection with a novel triple antimicrobial-bonded arterial graft. J Vasc Surg. 2016;64(6):1805–14.
14. Keidar Z, Nitecki S. FDG-PET in prosthetic graft infections. Semin Nucl Med. 2013;43(5):396–402.
15. Mitra A, Pencharz D, Davis M, Wagner T. Determining the diagnostic value of 18F-Fluorodeoxyglucose positron emission/computed tomography in detecting prosthetic aortic graft infection. Ann Vasc Surg. 2018;53:78–85.
16. Legout L, D'Elia PV, Sarraz-Bournet B, et al. Diagnosis and management of prosthetic vascular graft infections. Med Mal Infect. 2012;42(3):102–9.

17. Solomkin JS, Mazuski J, Blanchard JC, et al. Introduction to the Centers for Disease Control and Prevention and the Healthcare Infection Control Practices Advisory Committee guideline for the prevention of surgical site infections. Surg Infect (Larchmt). 2017;18(4):385–93.
18. Borchardt RA, Tzizik D. Update on surgical site infections: the new CDC guidelines. JAAPA. 2018;31(4):52–4.
19. Berríos-Torres SI, Umscheid CA, Bratzler DW, et al. Centers for Disease Control and Prevention guideline for the prevention of surgical site infection, 2017. JAMA Surg. 2017;152(8):784–91. Erratum in: JAMA Surg. 2017;152(8):803.
20. Anderson DJ, Sexton DJ. Overview of control measures for prevention of surgical site infection in adults. UpToDate. 2022.
21. Calderwood MS, Anderson DJ, Bratzler DW, et al. Strategies to prevent surgical site infections in acute-care hospitals: 2022 update. Infect Control Hosp Epidemiol. 2023;44(5):695–720.
22. Inui T, Bandyk DF. Vascular surgical site infection: risk factors and preventive measures. Semin Vasc Surg. 2015;28(3–4):201–7.
23. Chirca I, Marculescu C. Prevention of infection in orthopedic prosthetic surgery. Infect Dis Clin North Am. 2017;31(2):253–63.
24. Segreti J, Parvizi J, Berbari E, et al. Introduction to the Centers for Disease Control and Prevention and Healthcare Infection Control Practices Advisory Committee guideline for prevention of surgical site infection: prosthetic joint arthroplasty section. Surg Infect (Larchmt). 2017;18(4):394–400.
25. Elens M, Dusoruth M, Astarci P, et al. Management and outcome of prosthetic vascular graft infections: a single center experience. Vasc Endovasc Surg. 2018;52(3):181–7.
26. Moussavian MR, Laschke MW, Schlachtenberger G, et al. Perigraft vascularization and incorporation of implanted Dacron prostheses are affected by rifampicin coating. J Vasc Surg. 2016;64(6):1815–24.
27. Kuehn C, Graf K, Mashaqi B, et al. Prevention of early vascular graft infection using regional antibiotic release. J Surg Res. 2010;164(1):e185–91.
28. Lawrence PF. Conservative treatment of aortic graft infection. Semin Vasc Surg. 2011;24(4):199–204.
29. Zamani N, Sharath SE, Barshes NR, et al. Long-term outcomes of lower extremity graft preservation using antibiotic beads in patients with early deep wound infections after major arterial reconstructions. J Vasc Surg. 2020;71(4):1315–21.
30. Igari K, Kudo T, Toyofuku T, et al. Treatment strategies for aortic and peripheral prosthetic graft infection. Surg Today. 2014;44(3):466–71.
31. Chakfé N, Diener H, Lejay A, et al. European Society for Vascular Surgery (ESVS) 2020 clinical practice guidelines on the management of vascular graft and endograft infections. Eur J Vasc Endovasc Surg. 2020;59(3):339–84. Erratum in: Eur J Vasc Endovasc Surg. 2020;60(6):958.
32. Laohapensang K, Arworn S, Orrapin S, et al. Management of the infected aortic endograft. Semin Vasc Surg. 2017;30(2–3):91–4.
33. Warren JA, Love M, Cobb WS, et al. Factors affecting salvage rate of infected prosthetic mesh. Am J Surg. 2020;220(3):751–6.
34. Rosen MJ, Bauer JJ, Harmaty M, et al. Multicenter, prospective, longitudinal study of the recurrence, surgical site infection, and quality of life after contaminated ventral hernia repair using biosynthetic absorbable mesh: the COBRA study. Ann Surg. 2017;265(1):205–11.
35. Rosen MJ, Krpata DM, Petro CC, et al. Biologic vs synthetic mesh for single-stage repair of contaminated ventral hernias: a randomized clinical trial. JAMA Surg. 2022;157(4):293–301.
36. Jacombs ASW, Karatassas A, Klosterhalfen B, et al. Biofilms and effective porosity of hernia mesh: are they silent assassins? Hernia. 2020;24(1):197–204.

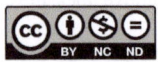

Surgical Wounds: Principles of Postoperative Care

16

Domitilla Foghetti

A surgical wound complication has considerable impact on the patient's quality of life and the wider healthcare setting [1] and it remains a significant challenge for clinicians as one of the leading causes of morbidity. Proper postoperative management of surgical wounds can reduce surgical site infection (SSI) rates, although patient-related risk factors, type of surgery and surgical technique are all components of a holistic assessment process.

16.1 Surgical Wound Management

In acute wounds, such as surgical skin incisions, an atmosphere with a proper moisture balance promotes cell migration and matrix formation, leading to complete healing 40% faster than a wound exposed to air. A suitable sterile dressing applied with an aseptic technique can absorb exudate, protect the wound from external environmental contamination, reduce tenderness and pain, and produce better cosmetic outcome [2, 3]. A 2015 Cochrane review showed no significant differences in SSI rates between early or delayed dressing removal from clean or clean-contaminated surgical wounds (low quality evidence) [4]. International guidelines suggest avoiding unnecessary touching of the wound site for at least 48 h after surgery, unless leakage or signs or symptoms of infection appear [4, 5]. It is recommended to wear gloves and to use the non-touch aseptic technique for removing or changing wound dressings; sterile saline can be used for wound cleansing up to 48 h after surgery, after which tap water is indicated and the patients may shower safely. Antiseptic agents should be considered for cleaning wounds that are infected [6].

D. Foghetti (✉)
Department of General Surgery, San Salvatore Hospital-AST Pesaro-Urbino, Pesaro, Italy
e-mail: domitilla.foghetti@gmail.com

S. Bartoli et al. (eds.), *Infections in Surgery*, Updates in Surgery,
https://doi.org/10.1007/978-3-031-60462-1_16

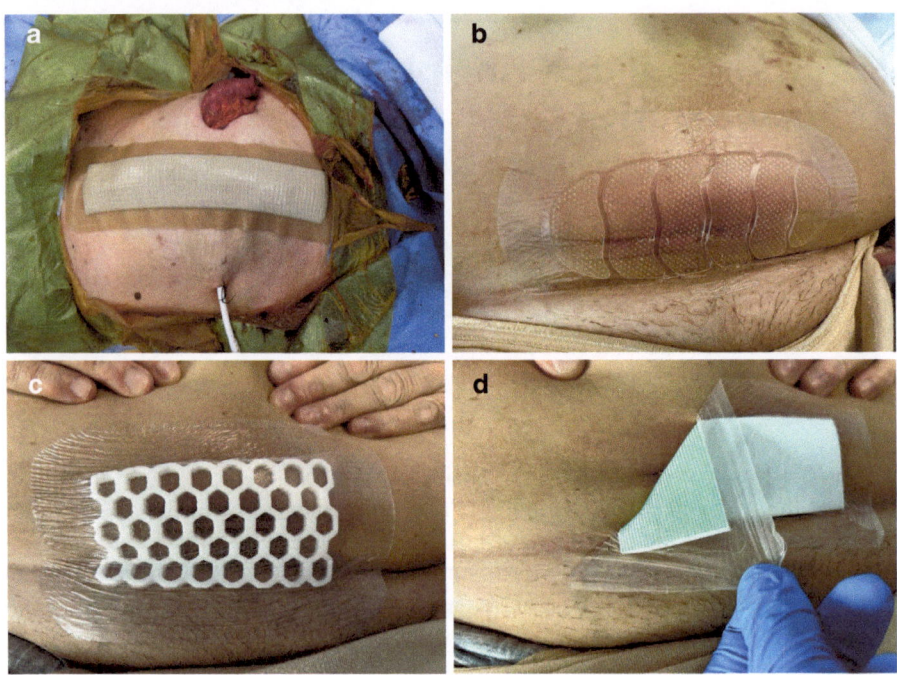

Fig. 16.1 (**a**) Multilayer post-surgical dressing with a mix of skin-friendly hydrocolloid technology and hydrofiber soft absorbent layer with ionic silver, covered with a polyurethane film that provides a waterproof and microorganism barrier. It can be used with a contemporary ostomy to protect the wound from external contamination. (**b**) Highly flexible and conformable transparent dressing, permeable only to air and water vapor, prevents skin maceration, protecting the wound against bacteria and viruses. (**c**) Semi-transparent surgical dressing can handle a small quantity of exudate, facilitates monitoring of the surgical site for early signs of infection while helping to maintain optimal wound moisture, protect skin integrity and prevent bacterial contamination; the low adherent wound contact layer helps to minimize pain on dressing removal. (**d**) Dialkylcarbamoyl chloride (DACC)-coated wound dressing manages wound microorganism bioburden by means of hydrophobic binding between the dressing and bacteria/yeast cells

Many different dressing types are available, but it is still unclear whether any one dressing is better than the other [5]. The ideal dressing should absorb and contain exudate, provide protection from the external environment (fluids, microorganisms) and thermal insulation, be transparent and flexible, guarantee patient comfort and absence of pain on removal, ensure a good cosmetic scar result, as well as being inexpensive. A 2016 Cochrane Review examined studies that compared a standard absorbent gauze with different interactive dressings (films, hydrocolloids, polyurethane matrix, hydroactive and antimicrobial dressings): the placement of any type of advanced dressing on primarily closed surgical wounds with the aim of preventing infection cannot be suggested (strength of the recommendation: conditional) [5–7]. Despite this, in 2019 the National Institute for Health and Care Excellence (NICE) published a guideline about SSI prevention, which suggests covering surgical incisions with an appropriate interactive dressing [8] (Fig. 16.1).

16.2 Topical Antibiotics and Antiseptic Agents

Topical antibiotics in the form of ointments, creams, gels or impregnated dressings applied after wound closure can reduce the risk of SSI (moderate quality of evidence) [9]. Their use remains controversial and the NICE 2019 guidelines do not suggest their routine use [8]. The relative effects of different antibiotics are unclear [10] and no definitive data are available about allergic contact dermatitis or impact on antibiotic resistance development. Topical antiseptic agents should be preferred over antibiotic agents, due to their broader spectrum of activity.

16.3 Surgical Wound Drainage

There is a paucity of evidence supporting the benefits of surgical wound drainage, even though different variables must be considered, such as type of surgery, patient-related risk factors, extent and location of surgery and potential microbiological burden. Its routine use does not seem to reduce the risk of SSI, but it can be useful in high-risk situations, such as obese patients or contaminated wounds [11]. The drain insertion site should be kept clean and covered with an appropriate dressing, and the skin must be inspected to detect signs of infection. To reduce the risk of SSI, drains should exit the skin away from the suture line and should be removed as soon as possible.

16.4 Incisional Negative Pressure Wound Therapy

Evidence of the effectiveness of incisional negative pressure wound therapy (iNPWT) single-use devices applied on closed surgical wounds to prevent surgical wound complications is accumulating in orthopedic [12], abdominal [13], vascular [14], cardiothoracic [15], obstetric, plastic/breast, and trauma surgery. Their pump is smaller, lighter and more portable than the conventional devices and the dressing system (peel-and-place or customizable) is easier to apply and remove, allowing for greater utilization [16]. The negative pressure level is maintained between −75 and −125 mmHg on the wound surface and exudate can be managed predominantly by evaporation in a canister-free system (Fig. 16.2) or collection in a small canister (Fig. 16.3). Clinical experiences reported that iNPWT reduces lateral tension on the incision line, increases blood flow and decreases edema [17, 18]. Even though its role remains uncertain in terms of reducing the incidence of seroma/hematoma, wound dehiscence and wound-related readmission to hospital within 30 days [19], the use of iNPWT is associated with a reduction in SSI rates [20, 21], especially in general and colorectal surgery [22].

The World Health Organization *Global guidelines for the prevention of surgical site infection* recommend the use of prophylactic NPWT on surgical incisions only in high-risk wounds, taking into account the available resources (conditional recommendation, low quality evidence) [7]. Surgical risk

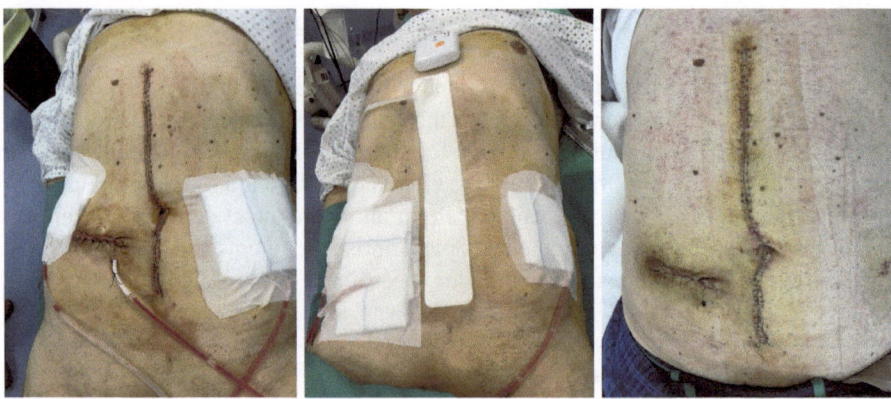

Fig. 16.2 Incisional negative pressure wound therapy: canister-less single-use device. Postoperative application in laparotomy for stoma reversal in a high-risk patient. The wound contact layer is a perforate flexible silicone, bonded to a lower airlock layer and an upper fluid absorption layer that delivers negative pressure, removes wound exudate and aids fluid evaporation through a highly breathable film layer. In high-risk surgical incisions, the device helps to reduce lateral tensile forces and increase the activity of the lymphatic system in deep tissues. It delivers continuous negative pressure at −80 mmHg. The dressing can be removed 7 days after surgery

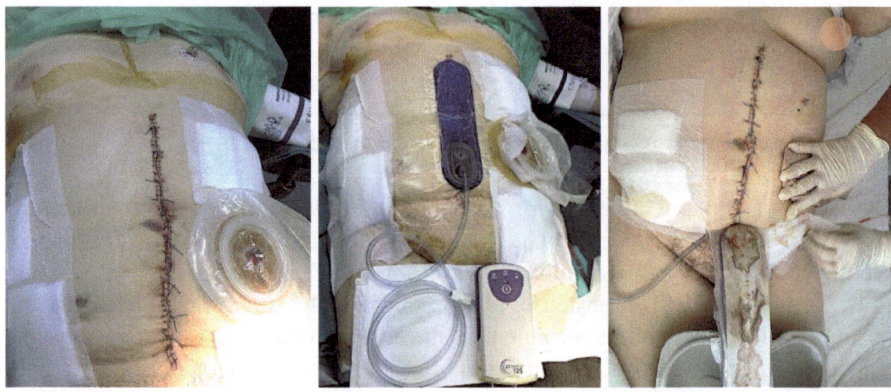

Fig. 16.3 Incisional negative pressure wound therapy: single-use device with a small canister. The device is available as a peel-and-place or customizable dressing in polyurethane foam, with ionic silver in the skin interface layer. It acts as a barrier to external contamination and delivers continuous negative pressure at −125 mmHg up to 7 days to the incision line. The single-use 45 mL canister is replaceable

calculators were developed to identify high risk patients based on the results of preoperative assessment (ASA score), surgical wound classification (from clean to dirty-infected) and duration of operation (National Nosocomial Infection

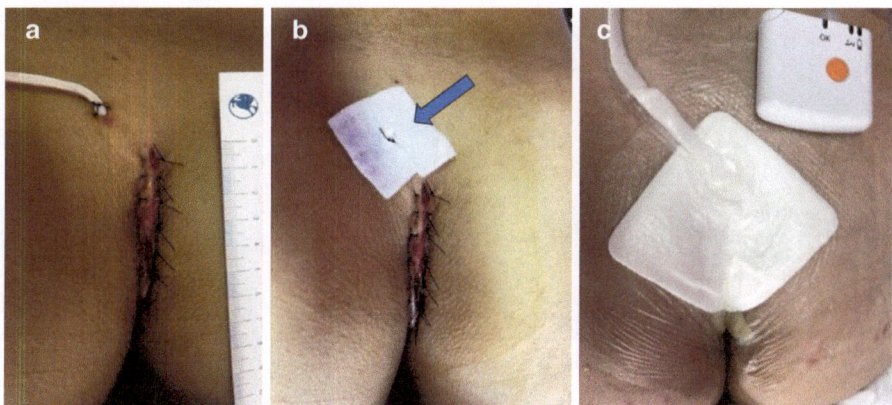

Fig. 16.4 (**a**) Surgical wound closed by primary intention after pilonidal cyst removal, with subcutaneous suction drain. (**b**) Surgical drain cut 1 cm from the skin 3 days after surgery. (**c**) Incisional negative pressure wound therapy applied over the subcutaneous drain and surgical wound. This prevents serum collection in the subcutaneous tissue, which is associated with infection and wound dehiscence. The dressing and drain can be removed after 7 days. If necessary, a 14-day device is also available

Surveillance Risk Index, NNIS) [23]. Surgical wounds such as sternotomies [15], laparotomies for ventral hernia repair [24], major limb amputations [25], perineal wounds in abdominoperineal resection for rectal cancer [26], reversals of temporary stomas [27] and pilonidal cyst removals are considered high risk surgical wounds.

Before surgery, the site of incision of any stomas and drains must be evaluated to ensure correct accommodation of an iNPWT dressing. To avoid blood or serum collecting in subincisional tissue, associated with a major risk of infection or dehiscence, a subcutaneous drain can be placed in selected wounds; it can be cut 1–2 cm from the skin 3–4 days after surgery, and covered with the iNPWT dressing, which will be removed after 7 days (Fig. 16.4). If the peel-and-place or customizable dressing does not fit with a particular shape of surgical wound, it is possible to consider the conventional device with a gauze dressing, which can be modelled on the surgical line (Figs. 16.5 and 16.6).

Studies regarding the economic and organizational sustainability of iNPWT for SSI prevention are in progress [28] and aim to assess whether investing in prevention delivers advantages for patients and healthcare systems, considering the treatment costs that can be avoided (further dressings, laboratory or diagnostic examinations, length of hospital stay or readmission rate, antibiotic and analgesic drugs, etc.), the human suffering and social costs, and the delays in adjuvant therapies in oncological patients.

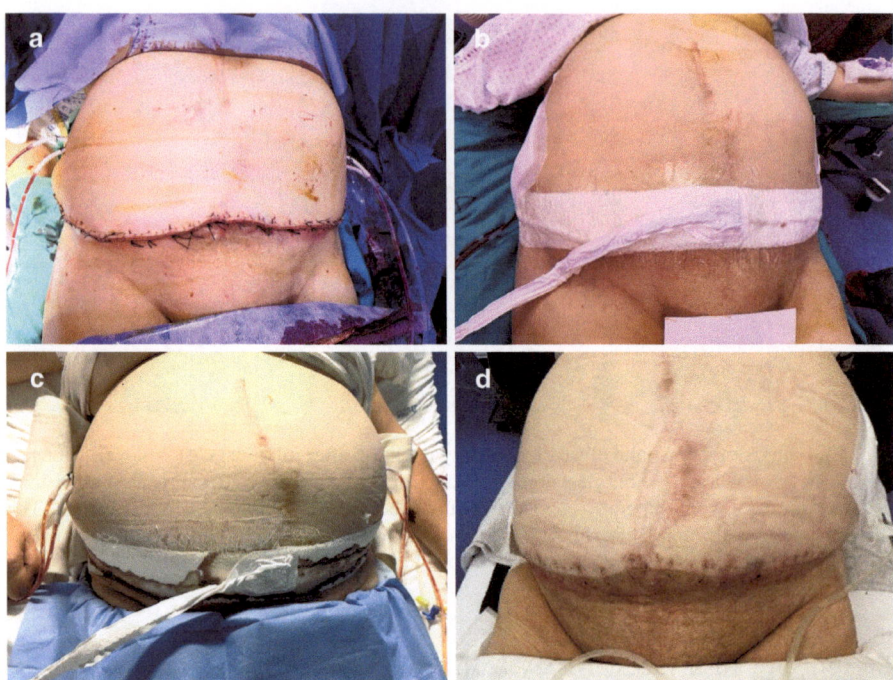

Fig. 16.5 After a high-risk procedure in high-risk patients, such as those who are obese, diabetic or smokers, conventional negative pressure wound therapy (NPWT) with gauze may be placed to reduce lateral tensile forces and subcutaneous edema. (**a**) Emergency surgery to repair a strangulated incisional hernia with abdominal wall skin necrosis and necessary abdominoplasty. (**b**) Conventional NPWT with gauze applied over the incisional wound. (**c**) Serum absorption by the gauze, before dressing removal after 5 days. (**d**) Completely healed surgical wound, without any complications, after removal of the stitches

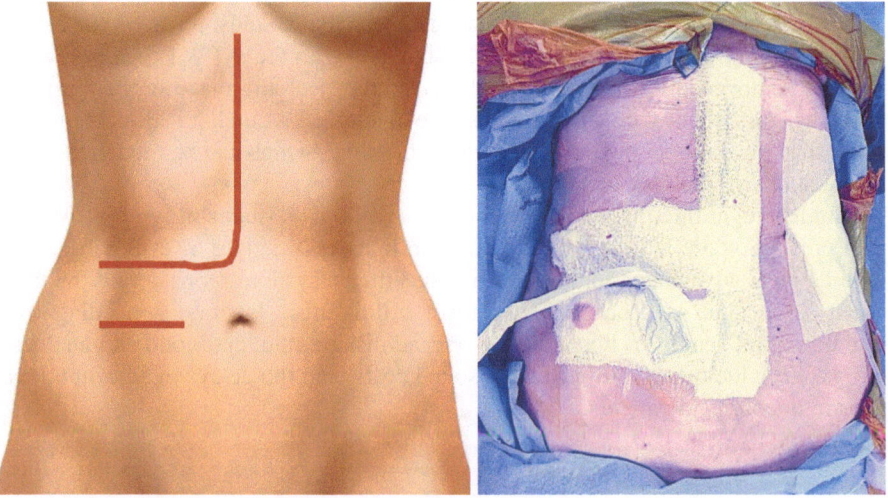

Fig. 16.6 Liver metastasectomy and ileostomy reversal in patient undergoing rectal resection for cancer with diverting ileostomy. Conventional negative pressure wound therapy (NPWT) with gauze was chosen to reduce infection and dehiscence risk in a patient with high-risk surgery and high-risk surgical site. A suction drain, cut at 1 cm from skin, was positioned in the subcutaneous tissue at the previous ileostomy site and covered with NPWT antibacterial gauze

16.5   Monitoring the Surgical Wound After Hospital Discharge

As a consequence of the reduction of postoperative hospitalization, the number of SSIs diagnosed postdischarge continues to rise. A large study in the US identified SSIs as the most common reason for readmission to hospital (19.5%) [18]. The improvement of postdischarge surveillance and the development of a high-quality homecare program can contribute to achieve an accurate and efficient system to better measure surgical outcomes and to estimate the human, social and financial impact of complications [29, 30]. A simple leaflet with information for patients regarding surgical wound care and numbers to contact a healthcare professional, if necessary, may be delivered, especially if the patient has an iNPWT device [31].

Direct patient contact, through a telephone survey or questionnaire at 30 days, can be used to collect data prospectively to calculate the SSI rates and improve the standards of care. A specialist wound care service should guarantee a structured approach to care to improve the management of surgical wounds [8]. Patients' experiences and feelings about surgical wounds and dressings are beginning to be considered by the surgical teams, even though the data produced from patient interviews need to be supplemented and integrated by further randomized controlled trials [32].

References

1. Conway B, McIsaac C, Tariq G, et al. Optimising prevention of surgical wound complications: detection, diagnosis, surveillance and prediction. ISWCAP (International Surgical Wound Complications Advisory Panel) international consensus document. London: Wounds International; 2022.
2. Delmore B, Cohen JM, Chu A, et al. Reducing postsurgical wound complication: a critical review. Adv Skin Wound Care. 2017;30(6):272–86.
3. Stryja J, Sandy-Hodgetts K, Collier M, et al. Surgical site infection: preventing and managing surgical site infection across health care sectors. J Wound Care. 2020;29(Sup 2b):S1–S72.
4. Toon CD, Lusuku C, Ramamoorthy R, et al. Early versus delayed dressing removal after primary closure of clean and clean-contaminated surgical wounds. Cochrane Database Syst Rev. 2015;2015(9):CD010259.
5. Dumville JC, Gray TA, Walter CJ, et al. Dressings for the prevention of surgical site infection. Cochrane Database Syst Rev. 2016;12(12):CD003091.
6. Milne J, Vowden P, Fumarola S, Leaper D. Postoperative incision management made easy. Wounds UK. 2012;8(suppl 4):1–4. https://wounds-uk.com/wp-content/uploads/sites/2/2023/02/content_10639.pdf. Accessed 16 Mar 2024
7. World Health Organization. Global guidelines for the prevention of surgical site infection. 2nd ed. Geneva: WHO; 2018. https://www.who.int/publications/i/item/9789241550475. Accessed 16 Mar 2024
8. NICE National Institute for Health and Care Excellence. Surgical site infections: prevention and treatment (NG125). Guideline 2019 (updated Aug 2020). https://www.nice.org.uk/guidance/ng125. Accessed 16 Mar 2024.
9. Heal CF, Banks JL, Lepper DP, et al. Topical antibiotics for preventing surgical site infection in wounds healing by primary intention. Cochrane Database Syst Rev. 2016;11(11):CD011426.
10. Banerjee S, Argáez C. Topical antibiotics for infection prevention: a review of the clinical effectiveness and guidelines. Ottawa, ON: Canadian Agency for Drugs and Technologies in Health; 2017. https://www.ncbi.nlm.nih.gov/books/NBK487430/. Accessed 16 Mar 2024

11. Manzoor B, Heywood N, Sharma A. Review of subcutaneous wound drainage in reducing surgical site infection after laparotomy. Surg Res Pract. 2015;2015:715803.
12. Karlakki S, Brem M, Giannini S, et al. Negative pressure wound therapy for management of the surgical incision in orthopaedic surgery: a review of evidence and mechanisms for an emerging indication. Bone Joint Res. 2013;2(12):276–84.
13. Sahebally SM, McKevitt K, Stephens I, et al. Negative pressure wound therapy for closed laparotomy incision in general and colorectal surgery: a systematic review and meta-analysis. JAMA Surg. 2018;153(11):e183467.
14. Pleger SP, Nink N, Elzien M, et al. Reduction of groin wound complications in vascular surgery patients using closed incision negative pressure therapy (ciNPT): a prospective, randomised, single-institution study. Int Wound J. 2018;15(1):75–83.
15. Atkins BZ, Wooten MK, Kistler J, et al. Does negative pressure wound therapy have a role in preventing poststernotomy wound complications? Surg Innov. 2009;16(2):140–6.
16. Malmsjö M, Huddleston E, Martin R. Biological effects of a disposable, canisterless negative pressure wound therapy system. Eplasty. 2014;14:e15.
17. Stannard JP, Gabriel A, Lehner B. Use of negative pressure wound therapy over clean, closed surgical incisions. Int Wound J. 2012;9(Suppl 1):32–9.
18. World Union of Wound Healing Societies (WUWHS). Consensus document. Close surgical incision management: understanding the role of NPWT. London: Wounds International; 2016.
19. Norman G, Shi C, Goh EL, et al. Negative pressure wound therapy for surgical wounds healing by primary closure. Cochrane Database Syst Rev. 2022;4(4):CD009261.
20. Hyldig N, Birke-Sorensen H, Kruse M, et al. Meta-analysis of negative-pressure wound therapy for closed surgical incisions. Br J Surg. 2016;103(5):477–86.
21. Sandy-Hodgetts K, Watts R. Effectiveness of negative pressure wound therapy/closed incision management in the prevention of post-surgical wound complications: a systematic review and meta-analysis. JBI Database System Rev Implement Rep. 2015;13(1):253–303.
22. Pellino G, Sciaudone G, Selvaggi F, Canonico S. Prophylactic negative pressure wound therapy in colorectal surgery. Effects on surgical site events: current status and call to action. Updat Surg. 2015;67(3):235–45.
23. Culver DH, Horan TC, Gaynes RP, et al. Surgical wound infection rates by wound class, operative procedure, and patient risk index. National Nosocomial Infections Surveillance System. Am J Med. 1991;91(3B):152S–7S.
24. Swanson EW, Cheng HT, Susarla SM, et al. Does negative pressure wound therapy applied to closed incisions following ventral hernia repair prevent wound complications and hernia recurrence? A systematic review and meta-analysis. Plast Surg (Oakv). 2016;24(2):113–8.
25. Zayan NE, West JM, Schulz SA, et al. Incisional negative pressure wound therapy: an effective tool for major limb amputation and amputation revision site closure. Adv Wound Care (New Rochelle). 2019;8(8):368–73.
26. Van der Valk MJM, De Graaf EJR, Doornebosch PG, Vermaas M. Incisional negative pressure wound therapy for perineal wounds after abdominoperineal resection for rectal cancer, a pilot study. Adv Wound Care (New Rochelle). 2017;6(12):425–9.
27. Poehnert D, Hadeler N, Schrem H, et al. Decreased superficial surgical site infections, shortened hospital stay, and improved quality of life due to incisional negative pressure wound therapy after reversal of double loop ileostomy. Wound Repair Regen. 2017;25(6):994–1001.
28. Foglia E, Ferrario L, Garagiola E, et al. Economic and organizational sustainability of a negative-pressure portable device for the prevention of surgical-site complications. Clinicoecon Outcomes Res. 2017;9:343–51.
29. Strugala V, Martin R. Meta-analysis of comparative trials evaluating a prophylactic single-use negative pressure wound therapy for the prevention of surgical site complications. Surg Infect (Larchmt). 2017;18(7):810–9.
30. Ingargiola MJ, Daniali LN, Lee ES. Does the application of incisional negative pressure therapy to high-risk wounds prevent surgical site complications? A systematic review. Eplasty. 2013;13:e49.

31. UK Health Security Agency. Monitoring surgical wounds for infection: information for patients. 2013 (updated Sep 2022). https://www.gov.uk/government/publications/monitoring-surgical-wounds-for-infection-information-for-patients. Accessed 16 Mar 2024.
32. Elliott D, Bluebelle Study Group. Developing outcome measures assessing wound management and patient experience: a mixed methods study. BMJ Open. 2017;7(11):e016155.

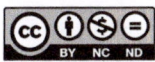

Critically Ill Surgical Patients in the Intensive Care Unit

17

Irene Coloretti and Massimo Girardis

17.1 Epidemiology of Intra-Abdominal Infection in the Intensive Care Unit

Intra-abdominal infections (IAIs) are a significant cause of intensive care unit (ICU) admission and are considered the second leading cause of sepsis and septic shock, following respiratory infection, in critically ill patients [1]. According to the 2022 report provided by the Italian Group for the Evaluation of Interventions in Intensive Care Medicine (https://giviti.marionegri.it/portfolio/prosafe/), among approximately 30,000 adult patients admitted to 117 Italian ICUs, around 20% of those admitted for sepsis had IAI, and more than half of these patients developed septic shock, with an overall mortality of about 30%. Critically ill patients with complicated IAI often require extensive supportive care due to multiple organ failure, leading to an extended stay in ICU [2]. However, advancements in medical knowledge and available treatments have improved survival rates for many patients who previously faced early refractory shock. Therefore, a growing number of patients are surviving the initial phase of sepsis and frequently develop a long-lasting critical illness characterized by persistent organ dysfunction and tissue catabolism, which is referred to as persistent inflammation, immunosuppression, and catabolism syndrome (PICS) [3].

I. Coloretti · M. Girardis (✉)
Anesthesia and Intensive Care Unit, University Hospital of Modena and University of Modena and Reggio Emilia, Modena, Italy
e-mail: irenecoloretti@gmail.com; girardis.massimo@unimore.it

17.2   Initial Management: Toward a Personalized Approach

The high mortality rate associated with complicated IAIs underscores the importance of prompt and effective management. The essential pillars of treatment include:

1. Early diagnosis: rapidly identifying and diagnosing IAIs is crucial for timely intervention; this involves a thorough clinical assessment, appropriate imaging studies, and laboratory tests to confirm the presence of infection and its severity.
2. Effective source control: effective source control is necessary to eliminate the infectious focus and prevent further spread of the infection.
3. Early appropriate antimicrobial therapy: empiric antibiotic therapy should be promptly initiated with molecules and dosages based on patient risk factors for difficult-to-treat microorganisms, available cultures, and clinical conditions.
4. Organ resuscitation with fluids and vasopressors: in patients with IAI and septic shock, adequate fluid resuscitation and vasopressor support should be provided to maintain tissue perfusion and prevent organ failure.

As in other septic patients, a personalized approach is highly recommended in patients with IAI [4]. To this aim, identifying patient phenotype may help tailor the interventions. The PIRO (predisposition, insult/infection, response, and organ dysfunction) score was proposed as a method to characterize septic patients by evaluating the underlying risk factors, the characteristics of the infectious event, the degree of organ dysfunction and dysregulation of the inflammatory response. The PIRO approach has been validated by several studies and was demonstrated to be closely related to mortality risk [5]. Translating the PIRO approach in critically ill patients with abdominal infection:

- *Predisposition*
- The evaluation of pre-existing diseases, the presence of immunosuppression, previous infections, and the type and length of surgery allows for defining the patient's immune status and capacity to respond to and eradicate the infection adequately.
- *Infection*
- The early identification of the site of infection and the infecting microorganisms is fundamental. Risk scores, previously available culture data, and specific biomarkers (e.g., 1,3-β-d-glucan) may orient the empiric choice of antibiotic while waiting for the microbiological results. Although without well-established evidence, the use of fast microbiology for early identification of microorganisms and their resistance patterns can further improve the appropriate treatment of patients with complicated IAI.
- *Response*
- Evaluating the immune and inflammatory response using specific biomarkers (e.g., endotoxin levels, lymphocyte count, immunoglobulin levels) allows for

identifying specific phenotypes as hyper- or hypoinflammatory profiles that may benefit from different approaches in adjunctive therapies.
- *Organ dysfunction*
- Among organ dysfunctions, the cardiovascular system is often involved in patients with complicated IAI, and resuscitation strategies must carefully evaluate the proper fluid volume and vasopressor dose to avoid overload or excessive vasoconstriction, which could cause intra-abdominal hypertension and low abdominal organ perfusion.

17.3 Late Management: The Worsening Patient

Patients with complicated IAIs showing either no improvement or a worsening after appropriate initial management is a challenging scenario requiring an experienced multidisciplinary team that should evaluate three domains: uncontrolled infection, uncontrolled inflammatory/immune response, and side effects of therapies.

17.3.1 Uncontrolled Infection

Uncontrolled infection is the most frequent reason for persisting or worsening inflammation and organ dysfunction in critically ill patients with IAIs. It could be sustained by inadequate source control, other sources of infection or inappropriate antibiotic therapy in terms of the molecule of choice and dose regimen.

Commonly used biomarkers such as C-reactive protein (CRP) and procalcitonin (PCT) may help identify this condition. PCT has been largely investigated in sepsis, demonstrating the ability to differentiate infectious from non-infectious systemic inflammatory response syndrome [6]. PCT was proposed to be more sensitive when compared to other biomarkers as an early indicator of uncontrolled infection after major surgery [7], especially when considering its dynamic changes rather than concentration itself [8]. The WSES/GAIS/SIS-E/WSIS/AAST guidelines proposed clinical pathways for patients with IAI, indicating PCT and CRP as laboratory markers to be considered for early diagnosis and antibiotic discontinuation [1]. A recently published meta-analysis evaluated the diagnostic accuracy of PCT as a diagnostic biomarker for postoperative infection/sepsis following major abdominal surgery in ten studies involving 1611 patients, with high heterogeneity among the included studies [9]. The authors concluded that PCT performs only moderately well as a diagnostic test for postoperative infection/sepsis, demonstrating limited pooled sensitivity (median 72%; 95% CI 66–78%) and specificity (median 62%; 95% CI 59–64%). Otherwise, serial PCT measurements seem to be accurate in evaluating the efficacy of treatments to eradicate the infection. In this setting, PCT has been proposed to guide the discontinuation of antibiotic therapy and was demonstrated to be cost-effective [10]. In the recent multicenter MOSES study, the authors investigated the role of an early decrease in PCT levels in predicting mortality [11]. Results showed that patients with an initial increase in PCT from baseline to day 1 had threefold higher mortality (29%) than patients with an initial PCT decrease, with mortality rates of 12%. Recent guidelines for the management of sepsis and septic shock provided by the Surviving Sepsis Campaign suggest using PCT and clinical evaluation to decide when to discontinue antimicrobials over clinical evaluation alone in patients with adequate source control (weak recommendation, low quality of evidence) [12].

A patient with complicated IAI is at high risk of developing secondary infections due to opportunistic pathogens, and, among these, fungal infections are frequent. The incidence of invasive *Candida* infection (ICI) in septic patients is increasing [13]. The mortality burden for these patients reaches 80% if no antifungal treatment is started within the first 24 h of septic shock [14]. Current guidelines suggest early antifungal treatment in critically ill patients with a high risk of ICI but contain few indications on selecting appropriate patients [12]. A recent report from the EUCANDICU project [13] showed a cumulative incidence of candidemia and ICI of 5.52 and 1.84 episodes per 1000 ICU admissions, with crude 30-day mortality significantly higher in candidemia/IAC patients. A fundamental easy-to-measure biomarker related to ICI is 1,3-β-d-glucan (BDG). BDG serum concentrations are elevated in patients with ICI [15]. Studies identified a cut-off value of 80 pg/mL to diagnose candidemia and abdominal candidiasis [16], even though higher specificity was achieved by elevating the cut-off to 200 pg/mL [17]. BDG performance was demonstrated to be superior to clinical prediction models and colonization indexes, showing in settings at low pretest probability (IC rate < 5%) high sensitivity (74–86%) and a negative predictive value >95% [18]. Due to these features, monitoring BDG in patients at risk of candidiasis has the role of ruling out the infection and de-escalating antifungal treatments [19]. A recent trial proposed a systematic approach in patients at high risk for ICI [20] suggesting that antifungal coverage may be appropriate, with re-assessment at 72–96 h. In the re-assessment, BDG levels of 80 pg/mL or lower and clinical stability should encourage antifungal de-escalation and ensure infection control. Otherwise, values of BDG between 80–200 pg/mL and clinical instability deserve further evaluation, and values above 200 pg/mL suggest ICI.

17.3.2 Uncontrolled Inflammatory/Immune Response

The research on pathobiological mechanisms of sepsis revealed a high heterogeneity of the inflammatory response [21], making it fundamental to identify the immune phenotype of each patient to personalize therapy. In recent years, several biomarkers have been proposed for detecting patients with immune failure and PICS, but, unfortunately, most of these are unsuitable for bedside use. Nevertheless, some easy-to-measure biomarkers may be rough but sound indicators of the efficiency of the immune response. For instance, HLA-DR expression on monocytes, lymphocyte count, neutrophil to lymphocyte ratio, and immunoglobulin plasma concentration are closely related to the risk of developing new infections and mortality in different critically ill patients with suspected immune dysfunction

[22]. Similarly, the reactivation of cytomegalovirus, Epstein-Barr virus, human herpesvirus 6, and herpes simplex virus, as well as infection by an opportunistic agent, such as *Acinetobacter* spp., *Enterococcus* spp., and *Candida* spp., have also been considered reliable and used for identification of an immunosuppressive pattern [23].

A specific cause of derangement of the immune system during IAI is the presence of endotoxemia. Endotoxin is a lipopolysaccharide composing the central part of the outer membrane of Gram-negative bacteria. Endotoxin is believed to be one of the principal mediators leading to organ dysfunction in patients with sepsis [24]. Furthermore, endotoxemia has been detected in patients with severe infections caused by Gram-positive bacteria and in critically ill patients with nonseptic conditions (e.g., trauma, cardiac surgery, burns), supporting the hypothesis of translocation from the gastrointestinal tract during critical illness [25]. High levels of endotoxin activity were found in critically ill patients admitted to the ICU with sepsis, and these levels were demonstrated to be closely related to the risk of developing organ dysfunction and poor outcome [26]. Recent innovations in blood purification techniques in sepsis moved from the broad clearance of humoral substances to the selective removal of identified targets involved in the immune-inflammatory response [27]. In this scenario, a cartridge with immobilized polymyxin B (PMX-B) was developed for extracorporeal hemoperfusion to remove endotoxin. In 2009, the Italian multicentre EUPHAS trial demonstrated in 64 patients with IAI undergoing emergency surgery that the early use of PMX-B hemoperfusion was associated with a reduction in the use of vasopressor drugs, and improvement in the Sequential Organ Failure Assessment (SOFA) score and 28-day mortality [28]. However, in 2015 the French multicenter ABDOMIX trial did not detect any difference in mortality and organ dysfunction in 243 patients with septic shock and peritonitis randomized to PMX-B hemoperfusion or placebo [29]. Similarly, a large retrospective observational study including 413 patients with septic shock and Gram-negative bacteria infection demonstrated no difference in 28-day mortality with the early use of PMX-B hemoperfusion [30]. This study was included in a systematic review and meta-analysis of 17 trials that outlined a correlation between patient severity and the effects obtained with PMX-B hemoperfusion, with a significant reduction of mortality in the intermediate- and high-risk groups, but not in the low-risk group [31]. The recently published multicenter EUPHRATES trial randomized 450 patients with refractory septic shock and high levels of endotoxin in the blood to receive standard treatment plus two PMX-B treatments (90–120 min) or sham treatment within 24 h of enrolment. PMX-B was not associated with a significant difference in mortality at 28 days among all patients or in the population with a multiple organ dysfunction score (MODS) >9 [32]. A post hoc analysis of the EUPHRATES trial showed that PMX-B seems to be effective in improving mortality and ventilator-free days in a specific population of patients with endotoxin activity measured between 0.6–0.89 [33]. The efficacy of blood purification in sepsis is still debated, and the evidence supporting its use is limited. The Surviving Sepsis Campaign's international guidelines for the management of sepsis and septic shock in 2021 [12] did not recommend the use of PMX-B hemoperfusion (weak recommendation; low quality of evidence), citing the lack of current evidence and the potential for significant costs of the technique to create inequity.

A patient experiencing a first episode of IAI with worsening clinical condition despite adequate source control and antibiotic therapy may be experiencing a dysregulated and/or persistent activation of the anti-inflammatory components, which may cause progressive immune exhaustion and lead to PICS. This immune failure is defined as immune paralysis and is characterized by impaired phagocytosis, alteration of the cytokine profile, inadequacy of antigen-presenting mechanisms, and dysfunction of B and T lymphocytes [22]. Patients with immune paralysis are unable to mount an effective inflammatory response and become prone to the persistence of infection, viral reactivation, and secondary or breakthrough infections, often by opportunistic agents such as *Acinetobacter* spp. and *Candida* spp. [34]. The elderly population, patients with nosocomial infections, comorbidities such as diabetes, and previous immunosuppression frequently show blunted inflammatory response and a predominant anti-inflammatory pattern [35].

17.3.3 Side Effects of Therapies

The side effects of therapies such as fluid therapy, vasoactive drugs, and antibiotics may be the cause of deterioration in critically ill patients with IAI. Fluid resuscitation is an essential part of the treatment of patients with sepsis and septic shock to counteract tissue hypoperfusion. Guidelines recommend initiating appropriate resuscitation immediately upon recognition of sepsis or septic shock as the best practice statement. The 2021 edition of the Surviving Sepsis Campaign guidelines recommends administering at least 30 mL/kg of intravenous crystalloid fluid within the first 3 h of resuscitation [12]. Especially in patients with intra-abdominal sepsis who underwent surgery, excessive fluid resuscitation may increase intra-abdominal pressure leading to intra-abdominal hypertension and worsening of the bowel edema, which is associated with a high risk of complications and worsening condition causing significant morbidity and mortality [36]. The effects of intra-abdominal hypertension on the gastrointestinal system are multiple and include mesenteric vein compression, abdominal and renal hypoperfusion, intestinal edema, bacterial translocation, and disruption of the gut microbiome with dysregulation of the immune system [37]. The risk factors for the development of intra-abdominal hypertension (such as abdominal surgery, ileus, gastric distention, IAI, massive fluid resuscitation, positive fluid balance, and shock [38]) are all present in complicated IAIs. Among these factors, the only factor that often can be avoided is excessive fluid resuscitation. It has been demonstrated that a higher volume of fluid during the first hours, but a lower volume in the 24 h, reduces mortality in severe sepsis and septic shock patients and that a positive total fluid balance increases mortality by 1.7 times [39]. Moreover, a positive fluid balance between 5 and 10 L in the first 48 h after damage-control laparotomy in 571 patients with an open abdomen was an independent risk factor for developing enteric fistula and abdominal sepsis

[40]. For these reasons, in recent decades, the fluid therapy approach shifted from massive fluid resuscitation to more restrictive strategies [41]. Permissive hypotension with small-volume resuscitation, allowing transient organ underperfusion, was introduced to manage several conditions such as hemorrhagic shock. In hemorrhagic shock, permissive hypotension (mean arterial pressure 50–60 mmHg) proved to be safe and reduced dilution of clotting factors, hypothermia, increase of hydrostatic pressure, and abdominal hypertension [42]. A recent randomized controlled trial compared a permissive hypotension (mean arterial pressure [MAP] 60–65 mm Hg) group with standard-of-care (MAP 75–80 mmHg) in 118 patients with septic shock [43]. The authors found reduced hospital mortality in older patients in the permissive hypotension group. In a further study, a total of 2463 patients with septic shock aged more than 65 years were included [44]; exposure to vasopressors was significantly less in the intervention group with target MAP 60–65 mmHg, and 90-day mortality in the two groups was similar (41.0 vs. 43.8%). This may introduce, even in septic shock patients, the concept of transient permissive hypotension and reduce the amount of fluids and vasopressors administered. The Conservative versus Liberal Approach to Fluid Therapy of Septic Shock in Intensive Care (CLASSIC) [45] and the Crystalloid Liberal or Vasopressors Early Resuscitation in Sepsis (CLOVERS) [46] trials were designed to address whether a restrictive versus a liberal fluid administration would improve outcomes in patients with sepsis and septic shock. In both trials, there was no difference in the primary outcome of 90-day mortality. Furthermore, a meta-analysis of studies evaluating a restrictive versus a liberal fluid strategy after initial resuscitation in sepsis demonstrated that the restrictive strategy was associated with a lower duration of mechanical ventilation but without effect on mortality [47].

17.4 Conclusions

In conclusion, critically ill patients with IAI remain a true challenge for intensivists, especially in situations of a lack of improvement and progressive worsening. Personalization of care is crucial for coping with individual patients' specific needs and it may be achieved by recognizing the diverse factors influencing a patient's immune response, including age, comorbidities, and genetic predisposition. A tailored approach extends beyond administering antibiotics and surgical interventions; it encompasses thoughtful consideration of resuscitative treatments, immunomodulatory therapies, and specific supportive measures. An in-depth exploration of the immune response should be considered in IAI patients, and the complexity of immune dysregulation requires a meticulous approach to patient care that goes beyond a "one-size-fits-all" treatment strategy. Finally, it is crucial to underscore the significance of interdisciplinary collaboration in managing critically ill patients with IAI. A seamless integration of expertise from infectious disease specialists, surgeons, immunologists, and intensivists fosters a holistic and comprehensive approach to patient care.

I. Coloretti and M. Girardis

References

1. Sartelli M, Coccolini F, Kluger Y, et al. WSES/GAIS/SIS-E/WSIS/AAST global clinical pathways for patients with intra-abdominal infections. World J Emerg Surg. 2021;16(1):49.
2. Cox MC, Brakenridge SC, Stortz JA, et al. Abdominal sepsis patients have a high incidence of chronic critical illness with dismal long-term outcomes. Am J Surg. 2020;220(6):1467–74.
3. Bergmann CB, Beckmann N, Salyer CE, et al. Lymphocyte immunosuppression and dysfunction contributing to persistent inflammation, immunosuppression, and catabolism syndrome (PICS). Shock. 2021;55(6):723–41.
4. Vincent JL, Singer M, Einav S, et al. Equilibrating SSC guidelines with individualized care. Crit Care. 2021;25(1):397.
5. Cardoso T, Rodrigues PP, Nunes C, et al. Prospective international validation of the predisposition, infection, response and organ dysfunction (PIRO) clinical staging system among intensive care and general ward patients. Ann Intensive Care. 2021;11(1):180.
6. Angeletti S, Battistoni F, Fioravanti M, et al. Procalcitonin and mid-regional pro-adrenomedullin test combination in sepsis diagnosis. Clin Chem Lab Med. 2013;51(5):1059–67.
7. Spoto S, Valeriani E, Caputo D, et al. The role of procalcitonin in the diagnosis of bacterial infection after major abdominal surgery: advantage from daily measurement. Medicine (Baltimore). 2018;97(3):e9496.
8. Guan J, Lin Z, Lue H. Dynamic change of procalcitonin, rather than concentration itself, is predictive of survival in septic shock patients when beyond 10 ng/mL. Shock. 2011;36(6):570–4.
9. Jerome E, McPhail MJ, Menon K. Diagnostic accuracy of procalcitonin and interleukin-6 for postoperative infection in major gastrointestinal surgery: a systematic review and meta-analysis. Ann R Coll Surg Engl. 2022;104(8):561–70.
10. Westwood M, Ramaekers B, Whiting P, et al. Procalcitonin testing to guide antibiotic therapy for the treatment of sepsis in intensive care settings and for suspected bacterial infection in emergency department settings: a systematic review and cost-effectiveness analysis. Health Technol Assess. 2015;19(96):v–xxv.
11. Schuetz P, Birkhahn R, Sherwin R, et al. Serial procalcitonin predicts mortality in severe sepsis patients: results from the Multicenter Procalcitonin MOnitoring SEpsis (MOSES) Study. Crit Care Med. 2017;45(5):781–9.
12. Evans L, Rhodes A, Alhazzani W, et al. Surviving sepsis campaign: international guidelines for management of sepsis and septic shock 2021. Crit Care Med. 2021;49(11):e1063–143.
13. Bassetti M, Giacobbe DR, Vena A, et al. Incidence and outcome of invasive candidiasis in intensive care units (ICUs) in Europe: results of the EUCANDICU project. Crit Care. 2019;23(1):219.
14. Kollef M, Micek S, Hampton N, et al. Septic shock attributed to Candida infection: importance of empiric therapy and source control. Clin Infect Dis. 2012;54(12):1739–46.
15. Ostrosky-Zeichner L, Alexander BD, Kett DH, et al. Multicenter clinical evaluation of the $(1\rightarrow3)$ β-D-glucan assay as an aid to diagnosis of fungal infections in humans. Clin Infect Dis. 2005;41(5):654–9.
16. Posteraro B, Tumbarello M, De Pascale G, et al. (1,3)-β-d-glucan-based antifungal treatment in critically ill adults at high risk of candidaemia: an observational study. J Antimicrob Chemother. 2016;71(8):2262–9.
17. León C, Ruiz-Santana S, Saavedra P, et al. Contribution of Candida biomarkers and DNA detection for the diagnosis of invasive candidiasis in ICU patients with severe abdominal conditions. Crit Care. 2016;20(1):149. Erratum in: Crit Care. 2017;21(1):107
18. Haydour Q, Hage CA, Carmona EM, et al. Diagnosis of fungal infections. A systematic review and meta-analysis supporting American Thoracic Society practice guideline. Ann Am Thorac Soc. 2019;16(9):1179–88.
19. Bailly S, Leroy O, Montravers P, et al. Antifungal de-escalation was not associated with adverse outcome in critically ill patients treated for invasive candidiasis: post hoc analyses of the AmarCAND2 study data. Intensive Care Med. 2015;41(11):1931–40.

20. De Pascale G, Posteraro B, D'Arrigo S, et al. (1,3)-β-D-glucan-based empirical antifungal interruption in suspected invasive candidiasis: a randomized trial. Crit Care. 2020;24(1):550.
21. Bosmann M, Ward PA. The inflammatory response in sepsis. Trends Immunol. 2013;34(3):129–36.
22. Hotchkiss RS, Monneret G, Payen D. Sepsis-induced immunosuppression: from cellular dysfunctions to immunotherapy. Nat Rev Immunol. 2013;13(12):862–74.
23. Ong DSY, Bonten MJM, Spitoni C, et al. Epidemiology of multiple herpes viremia in previously immunocompetent patients with septic shock. Clin Infect Dis. 2017;64(9):1204–10.
24. Cohen J. The detection and interpretation of endotoxaemia. Intensive Care Med. 2000;26(Suppl 1):S51–6.
25. Marshall JC, Foster D, Vincent JL, et al. Diagnostic and prognostic implications of endotoxemia in critical illness: results of the MEDIC study. J Infect Dis. 2004;190(3):527–34.
26. Biagioni E, Venturelli C, Klein DJ, et al. Endotoxin activity levels as a prediction tool for risk of deterioration in patients with sepsis not admitted to the intensive care unit: a pilot observational study. J Crit Care. 2013;28(5):612–7.
27. Di Carlo JV, Alexander SR. Hemofiltration for cytokine-driven illnesses: the mediator delivery hypothesis. Int J Artif Organs. 2005;28(8):777–86.
28. Cruz DN, Antonelli M, Fumagalli R, et al. Early use of polymyxin B hemoperfusion in abdominal septic shock: the EUPHAS randomized controlled trial. JAMA. 2009;301(23):2445–52.
29. Payen DM, Guilhot J, Launey Y, et al. Early use of polymyxin B hemoperfusion in patients with septic shock due to peritonitis: a multicenter randomized control trial. Intensive Care Med. 2015;41(6):975–84.
30. Saito N, Sugiyama K, Ohnuma T, et al. Efficacy of polymyxin B-immobilized fiber hemoperfusion for patients with septic shock caused by Gram-negative bacillus infection. PLoS One. 2017;12(3):e0173633.
31. Chang T, Tu YK, Lee CT, et al. Effects of polymyxin B hemoperfusion on mortality in patients with severe sepsis and septic shock: a systemic review, meta-analysis update, and disease severity subgroup meta-analysis. Crit Care Med. 2017;45(8):e858–64.
32. Dellinger RP, Bagshaw SM, Antonelli M, et al. Effect of targeted polymyxin B Hemoperfusion on 28-day mortality in patients with septic shock and elevated endotoxin level: the EUPHRATES randomized clinical trial. JAMA. 2018;320(14):1455–63.
33. Klein DJ, Foster D, Walker PM, et al. Polymyxin B hemoperfusion in endotoxemic septic shock patients without extreme endotoxemia: a post hoc analysis of the EUPHRATES trial. Intensive Care Med. 2018;44(12):2205–12.
34. Torgersen C, Moser P, Luckner G, et al. Macroscopic postmortem findings in 235 surgical intensive care patients with sepsis. Anesth Analg. 2009;108(6):1841–7.
35. Otto GP, Sossdorf M, Claus RA, et al. The late phase of sepsis is characterized by an increased microbiological burden and death rate. Crit Care. 2011;15(4):R183.
36. Bodnar Z. Polycompartment syndrome—intra-abdominal pressure measurement. Anaesthesiol Intensive Ther. 2019;51(4):316–22.
37. Druml W. Intestinaler crosstalk: Der Darm als motor des multiorganversagens [Intestinal cross-talk: the gut as motor of multiple organ failure]. Med Klin Intensivmed Notfmed. 2018;113(6):470–7.
38. Kirkpatrick AW, Roberts DJ, De Waele J, et al. Intra-abdominal hypertension and the abdominal compartment syndrome: updated consensus definitions and clinical practice guidelines from the world Society of the Abdominal Compartment Syndrome. Intensive Care Med. 2013;39(7):1190–206.
39. Tigabu BM, Davari M, Kebriaeezadeh A, Mojtahedzadeh M. Fluid volume, fluid balance and patient outcome in severe sepsis and septic shock: a systematic review. J Crit Care. 2018;48:153–9.
40. Bradley MJ, Dubose JJ, Scalea TM, et al. Independent predictors of enteric fistula and abdominal sepsis after damage control laparotomy: results from the prospective AAST Open Abdomen registry. JAMA Surg. 2013;148(10):947–54.

41. Boyd JH, Forbes J, Nakada TA, et al. Fluid resuscitation in septic shock: a positive fluid balance and elevated central venous pressure are associated with increased mortality. Crit Care Med. 2011;39(2):259–65.
42. Spahn DR, Bouillon B, Cerny V, et al. The European guideline on management of major bleeding and coagulopathy following trauma: fifth edition. Crit Care. 2019;23(1):98.
43. Lamontagne F, Meade MO, Hébert PC, et al. Higher versus lower blood pressure targets for vasopressor therapy in shock: a multicentre pilot randomized controlled trial. Intensive Care Med. 2016;42(4):542–50.
44. Lamontagne F, Richards-Belle A, Thomas K, et al. Effect of reduced exposure to vasopressors on 90-day mortality in older critically ill patients with vasodilatory hypotension: a randomized clinical trial. JAMA. 2020;323(10):938–49.
45. Meyhoff TS, Hjortrup PB, Wetterslev J, et al. Restriction of intravenous fluid in ICU patients with septic shock. N Engl J Med. 2022;386(26):2459–70.
46. National Heart, Lung, and Blood Institute Prevention and Early Treatment of Acute Lung Injury Clinical Trials Network, Shapiro NI, Douglas IS, et al. Early restrictive or liberal fluid management for sepsis-induced hypotension. N Engl J Med. 2023;388(6):499–510.
47. Reynolds PM, Stefanos S, MacLaren R. Restrictive resuscitation in patients with sepsis and mortality: a systematic review and meta-analysis with trial sequential analysis. Pharmacotherapy. 2023;43(2):104–14.

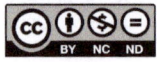

Synergy Between Infection Prevention and Control and Enhanced Recovery After Surgery

18

Felice Borghi, Luca Pellegrino, and Sara Salomone

18.1 ERAS Definition

ERAS, acronym of Enhanced Recovery After Surgery, is a multimodal perioperative pathway designed to reduce surgical stress for patients undergoing major surgery. Educating and enrolling patients in decision making, attention to optimal nutrition and pain control, and rapid return to the body's baseline functions are all common goals of this program.

The protocol, created by H. Kehlet for colon surgery in the '90 s, was previously called "fast-track surgery" and it is composed of several evidence-based elements that are individually effective in improving postoperative outcomes [1]. If used together, these elements—divided into preadmission, preoperative, intraoperative, and postoperative phases—have a synergic effect ensuring better results compared with the traditional perioperative care. Figure 18.1 shows the items of the ERAS protocol in colorectal surgery.

Since the different ERAS items are implemented by several medical and healthcare specialties a multidisciplinary approach is necessary. Because of the complexity of the program, the team should perform continuous audit of the care process and patient outcomes in order to make the necessary changes to improve the effectiveness of the pathway.

In 2010 the ERAS Society was officially registered as a not-for-profit medical society based in Stockholm with the mission of developing perioperative care and improving recovery of surgical patients through research, education, audit and implementation of evidence-based practice. In the last 10 years several new and updated guidelines have been published in different surgical fields and are available on the official ERAS website (https://erassociety.org).

F. Borghi (✉) · L. Pellegrino · S. Salomone
Surgical Department and Oncologic Surgery Unit, Candiolo Cancer
Institute, FPO-IRCCS, Candiolo (Turin), Italy
e-mail: felice.borghi@ircc.it; luca.pellegrino@ircc.it; sara.salomone@ircc.it

© The Author(s) 2025   153
S. Bartoli et al. (eds.), *Infections in Surgery*, Updates in Surgery,
https://doi.org/10.1007/978-3-031-60462-1_18

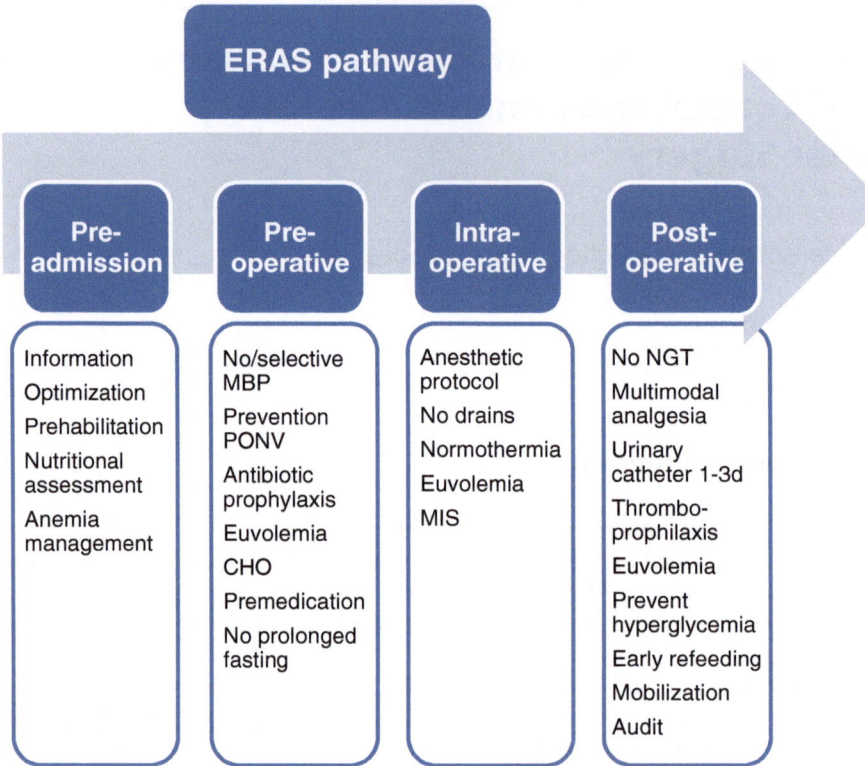

Fig. 18.1 Enhanced recovery after surgery (ERAS) items in colorectal surgery. *CHO* carbohydrate overloading; *MBP* mechanical bowel preparation; *MIS* minimally invasive surgery; *NGT* nasogastric tube; *PONV* postoperative nausea and vomiting

18.2 The Advantages of the ERAS Protocol

It is difficult to build comparative blinded studies between the ERAS protocol and traditional perioperative surgical care and, consequently, there is no uniformity in the published randomized trials. Moreover, the number of items used in each study is highly variable. Most of the available data concern colorectal surgery (CRS) for which, despite the drawbacks in the methodology and the weaknesses of meta-analyses, a 2–2.5-day reduction in length of stay (LOS) and a 30–50% reduction in complication rates compared to traditional care have been demonstrated [2].

Analysis of the ERAS international database for CRS shows that the better the compliance with the protocol, the better the outcomes with regard to both recovery time and complication rates. Probably a cut-off of >70% in adherence must be reached to achieve the favorable results of the ERAS protocol [3].

Greco et al., in a meta-analysis of 16 randomized clinical trials including 2376 patients, report that the ERAS pathway reduces primary nonsurgical complications, especially cardiopulmonary, rather than surgical complications [2]. If surgical complications and anastomotic leaks are mainly linked to patient-related factors or caused by technical shortcomings, probably they are only slightly modified by the ERAS pathways. Among the surgical complications, surgical site infections (SSIs) are the most common hospital-acquired infection in Europe (21.6%) and the most frequent complication after surgical procedures, with rates of up to 20% reported for CRS. Anastomotic leakage is one of the most feared surgical complications and is classified as an organ-space SSI. It is a serious postoperative infection that involves an increased risk of postoperative mortality and oncological recurrences, with worse survival of patients.

A significant financial burden, prolonged hospitalization, and higher consumption of antibiotic agents are associated with postoperative infection. The role of the ERAS pathway in reducing and preventing these complications is still unclear.

In a study performed by Gronnier et al. on 397 patients undergoing colonic surgery, the ERAS pathway and >70% compliance to ERAS items had no independent impact on SSI, while minimally invasive surgery (MIS) emerged as a protective factor for SSI [4]. Similar results were confirmed in our study on implementation of the ERAS pathway in the Piedmont region, where no differences were recorded in terms of SSI and overall complications before and after the ERAS pathway was implemented in CRS, albeit with the limitation of suboptimal compliance [5].

On the other hand, the POWER (Postoperative Outcomes Within Enhanced Recovery After Surgery Protocol) study, a multicenter trial including 80 Spanish hospitals and 2084 consecutive adults scheduled for elective CRS who either received or did not receive care in a self-declared ERAS center, showed that the number of patients with moderate or severe complications was lower in the ERAS group (25.2% vs. 30.3%). ERAS patients with highest adherence (>77%) compared to patients with lowest adherence (<54%) have fewer postoperative infections, including both superficial and deep SSI, but similar organ-space infections [6]. In some recent colorectal trials, the oncological results as well were found to be influenced by ERAS adherence, probably because the higher compliance group develops fewer complications that are strongly associated with poor long-term results [7].

To validate the importance of achieving optimal compliance, the reappraisal of the iCral2 and iCral3 prospective multicenter studies on CRS showed that the incidence of SSI, urinary tract, and pulmonary infections decreased from 7.7% to 3.0% with of adherence rates <55% or >85%, respectively [8].

Considering the general advantages in CRS, the ERAS protocol was also introduced with specific modifications by other different specialties. Currently, there are ERAS guidelines also for gastrectomy, esophagectomy, bariatric surgery, breast reconstruction, liver surgery, pancreaticoduodenectomy, emergency surgery, head and neck, orthopedic, cardiothoracic, gynecological, and urological surgery. Although most of the available literature concerns CRS, initial review studies in other areas of application of the ERAS program show similar benefits in short-term outcomes.

Grant et al., in a meta-analysis for abdominal or pelvic surgery, show a significant reduction in lung infection, urinary tract infection, and SSI when the ERAS pathway is applied. Also the subgroup analysis of the 18 trials involving only CRS and open incision studies confirmed a significant reduction in the same three outcomes for ERAS patients [9].

A recent meta-analysis, involving 4891 patients undergoing liver surgery, examined the impact of the ERAS program on wound infection, postoperative complications, and LOS. In this study, patient recovery was significantly reduced after implementation of ERAS but wound infections and complications were similar to those seen with traditional care [10].

The ERAS program is associated with shorter LOS, lower incidence of pulmonary complications, and reduction in hospital costs also for patients undergoing esophagogastric cancer surgery, but published studies have shown great heterogeneity and lack of definition of which ERAS elements were applied in each trial. Continuous monitoring of adherence is a crucial point to maintain and refine the ERAS protocol [11].

A meta-analysis supports the positive impact of the ERAS pathway on postoperative recovery after pancreatic duodenectomy, revealing significantly lower rates of abdominal infections and postoperative complications, and shorter LOS in the ERAS group [12]. A low compliance is related to higher postoperative complications, not only in CRS but also in pancreatic surgery. A recent trial aimed to assess the risk factors for SSI after pancreas surgery showing preoperative biliary stenting and male gender as the most relevant risk factors for developing SSI in the non-ERAS cohort, while no significant perioperative risk factors for SSI were found in the ERAS group. Moreover, a high compliance with the ERAS pathway is related to a lower incidence of SSI [13].

In Alberta (Canada), the healthcare service initially implemented an ERAS program for CRS that was subsequently extended across 9 hospitals to colorectal, pancreas, cystectomy, liver, and gynecologic oncology procedures. The health system savings per patient ranged from $26.35 to $3606.44, meaning that every dollar invested in ERAS would bring $1.05 to $7.31 in return. In CRS, a LOS reduction from 6 to 4½ days and an 11.7% reduction in complications leads to savings of $2806–$5898 per patient [14].

18.3 Integration of Postoperative Infection Prevention and ERAS Elements

The WHO published guidelines on interventions for the prevention of SSI that could be applied to all surgical specialties; these were followed by recommendations of other national institutions [15].

Many factors influence surgical wound healing and determine the potential risk for developing postoperative infections. These include patient-related and procedural-related variables. Some factors are obviously not modifiable, such as age and gender. However, other potential elements can be improved to reduce the likelihood of developing SSI and are often combined into different care bundles with the aim of improving compliance and enforcing their potential cumulative effect: avoiding razors for hair removal, limiting use of central venous catheters, maintaining normothermia, using of chlorhexidine gluconate plus alcohol-based skin preparation agents, performing intranasal decolonization, using anti-staphylococcal skin antiseptics for high-risk procedures, and using negative pressure wound therapy. Other factors such as nutritional status, tobacco use, preoperative optimization, correct use of antibiotics, fluid management, normothermia, use of MIS, and controlling for perioperative glucose concentrations are elements of the ERAS pathway that influence the development of postoperative infections. The role of integrating the ERAS pathway and SSI care bundles is difficult to assess owing to the gap between best scientific evidence and clinical practice. Elsewhere care bundles vary between different protocols, and the degree to which each plays a role in reducing SSI remains difficult to determine.

18.3.1 Which Elements of the Preadmission Phase of the ERAS Pathway Can Reduce Postoperative Infections?

Prehabilitation is a novel concept referring to preparing patients preoperatively to withstand the challenges of surgical stress, especially for those with comorbidities and frailty. The preoperative time is a teachable moment where patients may improve their healthcare. There are many areas of prehabilitation: physical exercise/optimization, and nutritional and psychological support. Emerging evidence suggests benefits before major abdominal and cardiothoracic surgery in terms of reduced overall complications, especially cardiac complications and pulmonary infections. However, randomized studies are needed to confirm the role of prehabilitation for specific patients and surgical procedures within the ERAS program.

One of the fields of preoperative optimization is smoking cessation. Systematic reviews and meta-analyses comparing smokers with nonsmokers in elective surgery show that the risk of SSI is nearly doubled in active smokers. Smoking cessation 4 weeks before elective surgery is recommended by multiple societies and should be pursued in all patients [16].

Malnutrition leads to alterations in host immunity and makes patients more susceptible to postoperative infections. Early nutritional support can decrease the incidence of infectious complications in selected malnourished patients undergoing major surgery. Immunonutrition can play a role in many gastrointestinal, cardiac and spinal surgical procedures but the heterogeneity of published studies and their methodological limitations require further validation by additional high-quality studies with larger sample sizes [17].

Preoperative anemia is another cause of postoperative morbidity and mortality in patients undergoing major surgery. The iCral3 study, a prospective multicenter observational study on CRS performed in Italy, showed that perioperative blood transfusions are an independent risk factor for higher major morbidity and anastomotic leaks [18]. All patients scheduled for surgery should undergo preoperative screening to detect anemia and correct the hemoglobin concentration within a patient blood management approach, described in Chap. 20.

18.3.2 Which Elements of the Preoperative Phase of the ERAS Pathway Can Reduce Postoperative Infections?

Some measures, such as mechanical bowel preparation (MBP) and oral antibiotic (OA) prophylaxis, are specific CRS items and are used irregularly. Abandoned decades ago in colon surgery, MBP has recently experienced a resurgence in part due to a large retrospective series from the ACS-NSQIP registry showing benefit in reducing SSI [19]. Although there is wide agreement that antibiotic agents should be used prior to CRS, there is still debate as to whether they should be administered intravenously alone or combined with non-absorbable oral antimicrobial agents. The addition of OA to intravenous administration in patients undergoing MBP was shown to reduce the risk for SSI when compared with intravenous coverage alone or OA alone. However, a recent Cochrane review is more cautious as the evidence is limited by the quality of the studies performed [20]. Because no definitive evidence has been found on the equivalence of combined MBP plus OA with OA alone, a high-quality study with participants randomized to receive no preparation, OA alone, or a combination of MBP plus OA is needed to provide a definitive answer to this question. Both ERAS and SSI prevention guidelines recommend administration of antibiotic prophylaxis 30–60 min before the incision because the therapeutic tissue concentrations should be reached at the time of incision and maintained throughout the intervention [15, 21]. Excess duration is the most common error when using antibiotic prophylaxis and is associated with increased toxicity, costs, and bacterial resistance. Antibiotic delivery after wound closure does not decrease the risk of SSI.

18.3.3 Which Elements of the Intraoperative Phase of the ERAS Pathway Can Reduce Postoperative Infections?

Normothermia before and during surgery is maintained by combinations of forced warm air, skin warming, and warmed intravenous fluids. A recent systematic review shows that in noncardiac surgeries the use of active body surface warming systems is associated with lower rates of SSI and blood loss. Their use is strongly recommended in preventive infection guidelines in all procedures lasting more than 30 min [22].

MIS, including the robotic and laparoscopic approach, is associated with lower rates of SSI in several studies and in different surgical fields. Moreover, the combination of laparoscopy and the ERAS pathway is more beneficial in CRS for reducing LOS and short-term complications [23]. The ERAS guidelines recommend its use whenever the expertise is available and MIS is appropriate, with a strong recommendation grade [24]. The same applies to liver and gastric surgery, where MIS can improve postoperative morbidity. Regarding esophagectomy, a randomized study comparing MIS to open surgery shows a reduction in pulmonary infections from 34% to 12% for the MIS group [25]. Although MIS alone can improve the results, there is significant potential for further improvement in outcomes with adoption of the ERAS pathway.

18.3.4 Which Elements of the Postoperative Phase of the ERAS Pathway Can Reduce Postoperative Infections?

Postoperative hyperglycemia is associated with an increased risk of SSI in patients with and without diabetes, and strategies to prevent hyperglycemia are recommended in the guidelines. In a meta-analysis of 15 RCTs, the use of tight glycemic control (<150 mg/dL) compared to conventional control (>150 mg/dL) was associated with lower rates of SSI (9.4% vs. 16%) [26].

Early enteral refeeding together with the unnecessary insertion of central venous lines, and the early removal of urinary catheters are other instruments for reducing and preventing postoperative infection [17].

Audit is a crucial point of both the ERAS pathway and investigation into the prevention of postoperative infection. Periodic reports should be prepared and given to key stakeholders to provide feedback for monitoring results and adopting the corrective measures necessary to obtain the effectiveness of processes.

18.4   Conclusions

Postoperative infections are associated with longer hospital stays, higher complication rates, and greater costs. The ERAS program, by reducing surgical stress and enhancing the patient's recovery, decreases the likelihood of developing postoperative complications for patients undergoing major surgery. A multidisciplinary approach is key to improving adherence to the ERAS pathway and ensuring systematic adoption of the care bundles recommended by scientific societies as a means to prevent postoperative infection, thanks to the potential cumulative and synergistic effect of these two evidence-based pathways.

References

1. Kehlet H, Wilmore DW. Evidence-based surgical care and the evolution of fast-track surgery. Ann Surg. 2008;248(2):189–98.
2. Greco M, Capretti G, Beretta L, et al. Enhanced recovery program in colorectal surgery: a meta-analysis of randomized controlled trials. World J Surg. 2014;38(6):1531–41.
3. Gustafsson UO, Hausel J, Thorell A, et al. Adherence to the Enhanced Recovery After Surgery protocol and outcomes after colorectal cancer surgery. Arch Surg. 2011;146(5):571–7.
4. Gronnier C, Grass F, Petignat C, et al. Influence of enhanced recovery pathway on surgical site infection after colonic surgery. Gastroenterol Res Pract. 2017;2017:9015854–8.
5. Pagano E, Pellegrino L, Rinaldi F, et al. Implementation of the ERAS (Enhanced Recovery After Surgery) protocol for colorectal cancer surgery in the Piemonte Region with an Audit and Feedback approach: study protocol for a stepped wedge cluster randomised trial: a study of the EASY-NET project. BMJ Open. 2021;11(6):e047491.
6. Ripollés-Melchor J, Ramírez-Rodríguez JM, Casans-Francés R, et al. Association between use of Enhanced Recovery After Surgery protocol and postoperative complications in colorectal surgery: the Postoperative Outcomes Within Enhanced Recovery After Surgery Protocol (POWER) study. JAMA Surg. 2019;154(8):725–36. Erratum in: JAMA Surg. 2022;157(5):460
7. Pang Q, Duan L, Jiang Y, Liu H. Oncologic and long-term outcomes of Enhanced Recovery After Surgery in cancer surgeries—a systematic review. World J Surg Oncol. 2021;19(1):191.

8. Catarci M, Ruffo G, Viola MG, et al. High adherence to enhanced recovery pathway independently reduces major morbidity and mortality rates after colorectal surgery: a reappraisal of the iCral 2 and iCral 3 multicenter prospective studies. G Chir. 2023;43:e24.

9. Grant MC, Yang D, Wu CL, et al. Impact of enhanced recovery after surgery and fast track surgery pathways on healthcare-associated infections: results from a systematic review and meta-analysis. Ann Surg. 2017;265(1):68–79. Erratum in: Ann Surg. 2017;266(6):e123

10. Wang YL, Zhang FB, Zheng LE, et al. Enhanced recovery after surgery care to reduce surgical site wound infection and postoperative complications for patients undergoing liver surgery. Int Wound J. 2023;20(9):3540–9.

11. Triantafyllou T, Olson MT, Theodorou D, et al. Enhanced recovery pathways vs standard care pathways in esophageal cancer surgery: systematic review and meta-analysis. Esophagus. 2020;17(2):100–12.

12. Ji HB, Zhu WT, Wei Q, et al. Impact of enhanced recovery after surgery programs on pancreatic surgery: a meta-analysis. World J Gastroenterol. 2018;24(15):1666–78.

13. Joliat GR, Sauvain MO, Petermann D, et al. Surgical site infections after pancreatic surgery in the era of enhanced recovery protocols. Medicine (Baltimore). 2018;97(31):e11728.

14. Thanh N, Nelson A, Wang X, et al. Return on investment of the Enhanced Recovery After Surgery (ERAS) multiguideline, multisite implementation in Alberta. Canada Can J Surg. 2020;63(6):E542–50.

15. Allegranzi B, Bischoff P, de Jonge S, et al. New WHO recommendations on preoperative measures for surgical site infection prevention: an evidence-based global perspective. Lancet Infect Dis. 2016;16(12):e276–87.

16. Sørensen LT. Wound healing and infection in surgery: the pathophysiological impact of smoking, smoking cessation, and nicotine replacement therapy: a systematic review. Ann Surg. 2012;255(6):1069–79.

17. Xie J, Du Y, Tan Z, Tang H. Association between malnutrition and surgical site wound infection among spinal surgery patients: a meta-analysis. Int Wound J. 2023;20(10):4061–8.

18. Italian ColoRectal Anastomotic Leakage (iCral) Study Group. Patient-reported outcomes, return to intended oncological therapy and enhanced recovery pathways after colorectal surgery: a prospective multicenter observational investigation by the Italian ColoRectal Anastomotic Leakage (iCral 3) study group. Ann Surg Open. 2023;4:e267.

19. Scarborough JE, Mantyh CR, Sun Z, Migaly J. Combined mechanical and oral antibiotic bowel preparation reduces incisional surgical site infection and anastomotic leak rates after elective colorectal resection: an analysis of colectomy-targeted ACS NSQIP. Ann Surg. 2015;262(2):331–7.

20. Willis MA, Toews I, Soltau SL, et al. Preoperative combined mechanical and oral antibiotic bowel preparation for preventing complications in elective colorectal surgery. Cochrane Database Syst Rev. 2023;2(2):CD014909.

21. Gustafsson UO, Scott MJ, Hubner M, et al. Guidelines for perioperative care in elective colorectal surgery: Enhanced Recovery After Surgery (ERAS) Society recommendations: 2018. World J Surg. 2019;43(3):659–95.

22. Balki I, Khan JS, Staibano P, et al. Effect of perioperative active body surface warming systems on analgesic and clinical outcomes: a systematic review and meta-analysis of randomized controlled trials. Anesth Analg. 2020;131(5):1430–43.

23. Greer NL, Gunnar WP, Dahm P, et al. Enhanced recovery protocols for adults undergoing colorectal surgery: a systematic review and meta-analysis. Dis Colon Rectum. 2018;61(9):1108–18.

24. Ficari F, Borghi F, Catarci M, et al. Enhanced recovery pathways in colorectal surgery: a consensus paper by the Associazione Chirurghi Ospedalieri Italiani (ACOI) and the PeriOperative Italian Society (POIS). G Chir. 2019;40(4 Supp):1–40.

25. Biere SS, van Berge Henegouwen MI, Maas KW, et al. Minimally invasive versus open oesophagectomy for patients with oesophageal cancer: a multicentre, open-label, randomised controlled trial. Lancet. 2012;379(9829):1887–92.

26. Seidelman JL, Mantyh CR, Anderson DJ. Surgical site infection prevention: a review. JAMA. 2023;329(3):244–52.

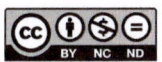

Patient Blood Management and Infection Prevention and Control

19

Marco Catarci, Michele Benedetti, Paolo Ciano, and Leonardo Antonio Montemurro

19.1 Introduction

Surgical site infections (SSIs) are the most common healthcare-associated infections following surgery and an important burden to inpatient surgery, with an incidence ranging from 2% to 5% of cases, a 2- to 11-fold increase in related mortality rates, prolonged hospitalization, and hospital readmissions [1]. Moreover, the development of SSIs has a significant impact on patient-reported outcomes and is a source of patient anxiety in the postoperative period, particularly after hospital discharge [2]. Patient blood management (PBM) is a multifactorial and multiprofessional bundle of evidence-based measures designed to maintain hemoglobin concentration and/or red cell mass, optimize hemostasis, minimize bleeding/blood loss during surgery, and enhance individual tolerance to postoperative anemia to avoid unnecessary blood transfusions and improve postoperative outcomes [3]. The aim of this chapter is to review the relationship between SSI and PBM based on the available evidence.

19.2 Perioperative Anemia, Blood Transfusions and Outcomes: The Hen-Egg Issue

Preoperative anemia, although generally considered a contraindication to elective surgery, is very common, affecting approximately one-third of patients who are candidates for general surgery [4], and nearly half of those undergoing colorectal, orthopedic and urologic procedures [5]. Logically, it is the strongest predictor of blood transfusions (fivefold) in the postoperative period, and, as a consequence, it is

M. Catarci (✉) · M. Benedetti · P. Ciano · L. A. Montemurro
Department of Surgery, Sandro Pertini Hospital, ASL Roma 2, Rome, Italy
e-mail: marco.catarci@aslroma2.it; michele.benedetti@aslroma2.it;
paolo.ciano@aslroma2.it; leonardo.montemurro@aslroma2.it

© The Author(s) 2025
S. Bartoli et al. (eds.), *Infections in Surgery*, Updates in Surgery,
https://doi.org/10.1007/978-3-031-60462-1_19

associated with several risks and morbidities, such as infections (twofold) and kidney injury (fourfold), as well as a 22% longer hospital stay. More importantly, perioperative anemia is now recognized as strongly and independently related to postoperative mortality (adjusted odds ratio 2.36), also independent of blood transfusions [6, 7]. Postoperative anemia occurs in up to 90% of patients after major surgery [8]. The main recognized causes are preoperative anemia, perioperative blood loss, poor nutritional intake in the postoperative period, frequent blood sampling for laboratory tests, and increased hepcidin due to inflammatory response to surgery. These effects can last for a few weeks after major surgery and aggravate postoperative iron deficiency anemia. Blood transfusions are the most widely used treatment for postoperative anemia. Blood transfusions carry several complications, culminating in a high incidence of morbidity and mortality [9–13]. In particular, they are related to increased length of hospital stay and rate of discharge to an inpatient facility, worse surgical and medical outcomes, allergic reactions, transfusion-related acute lung injury (TRALI), fluid overload, venous thromboembolism, graft-versus-host disease, immunosuppression, and postoperative infections. In addition, blood transfusions are responsible for increasing the burden on the healthcare system. Although the relationship between blood transfusion and poorer outcomes is not new, a clear understanding of the mechanism by which perioperative blood transfusions may worsen outcomes after surgery is still lacking. Apart from the long-standing and updated concept of transfusion-related immunomodulation (TRIM) and transient immunosuppression [14, 15], a recent retrospective propensity score-matched study of colorectal cancer surgery patients [16] suggested that worst early outcomes after surgery for colorectal cancer may be mediated by an exaggerated perioperative systemic inflammatory response in patients receiving perioperative blood transfusions. Moreover, recent experimental evidence [17] suggests a direct link between the gut flora composition (microbiota) and the development of antibody-mediated TRALI in mice. The recent introduction of metabolomics and proteomics to transfusion medicine [18] will possibly clarify how the microbiome and gut microbiota can affect the immune system shaping the antigenicity and contributing to TRIM and potential transmission of infection by blood donors.

However, the hen-egg issue regarding the relationship between perioperative blood transfusions and outcomes is still unsolved. It is still unclear if blood transfusions are a definite risk factor for poorer outcomes rather than a marker of bad performers: on the one hand, as reported above, perioperative blood transfusions may act directly by TRALI, TRIM, inflammatory response, and gut microbiome interactions; on the other hand, blood transfusions are generally more frequently administered in patients with major comorbidities, more extensive and longer procedures, more advanced cancer stages, and higher intraoperative blood loss. A recent propensity score-matched analysis of the iCral3 prospective multicenter observational study on colorectal surgery in Italy [13] showed that perioperative blood transfusions are an independent risk factor for higher major morbidity and anastomotic leakage rates, with 6 and 12 patients needed to avoid one major adverse event and one anastomotic leakage, respectively. While the majority of intra- and postoperative blood transfusions (IPBT) were administered as a consequence of intraoperative blood loss, postoperative hemorrhage and/or a postoperative major adverse event, in a small (5%) subgroup of patients IPBT preceded the major adverse event without any previous hemorrhagic event, showing the highest rates of adverse outcomes. It could be inferred, therefore, that improving transfusion appropriateness and eliminating this small subgroup of patients may allow a significant improvement of the outcomes. This is the main target of the recent calls for the urgent implementation of PBM programs [3, 19].

19.3 Patient Blood Management and Infection Prevention

In recent years, various strategies have been studied to reduce the use of blood transfusions to prevent transfusion-related adverse events, increase patient safety, and reduce costs. As a consequence, a new concept was born: PBM. According to the World Health Organization, PBM is defined as the timely application of evidence-based medical and surgical concepts designed to maintain a patient's hemoglobin concentration, optimize hemostasis, and minimize blood loss in an effort to improve the outcome [3]. More in detail, PBM focuses on three pillars: (a) optimizing red cell mass; (b) minimizing blood loss and bleeding; (c) optimizing tolerance of anemia. Implementation of the three pillars of PBM leads to improved patient outcomes by relying on his/her own blood rather than on that of a donor. PBM goes beyond the concept of appropriate use of blood products, because it precedes and strongly reduces the use of transfusions by correcting modifiable risk factors long before a transfusion may even be considered. Importantly, PBM is transversal to diseases, procedures and disciplines. It is solely aimed at managing a patient's resource (i.e., his/her blood), shifting the attention from the blood component to the patient himself/herself. Pragmatically, PBM consists of different approaches according to the considered pillar and to the time with respect to surgery.

According to different studies, PBM is able to reduce mortality up to 68%, reoperation up to 43%, readmissions up to 43%, composite morbidity up to 41%, infection rate up to 80%, average length of stay by 16–33%, transfusion from 10% to 95%, and costs from 10% to 84% [20].

In contrast to this favorable view of the effects of PBM implementation on outcomes, others argue that it does not improve any outcome beyond the significant reduction in perioperative blood transfusions, and it is therefore not cost-effective [21]. In fact, restrictive versus liberal transfusion thresholds are associated with a reduced risk of blood transfusions in randomized controlled trials, do not significantly reduce the rate of overall healthcare-associated infections [22, 23] but do significantly reduce the risk of serious healthcare-associated infections [22]. It should be noticed, however, that transfusion thresholds just represent a part of the whole PBM bundle. A longer implementation experience with a similar multifactorial, multidisciplinary and evidence-based bundle of perioperative care, such as the Enhanced Recovery After Surgery (ERAS) pathway [24–27], clearly showed that the bundle acts as a whole, with higher (i.e., beyond 70%) program adherence rates being significantly related to better outcomes in a close dose-effect relationship (see

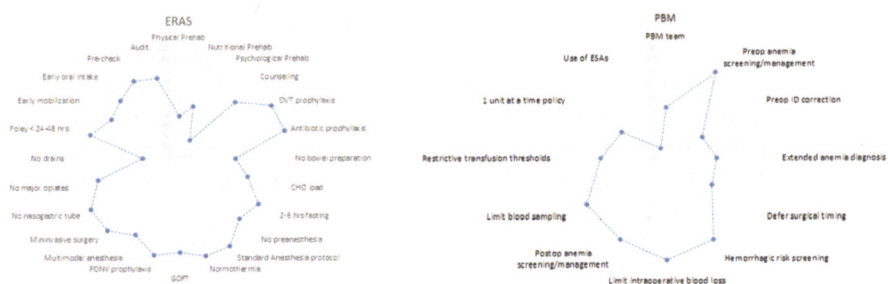

Fig. 19.1 Radar plot of adherence to enhanced recovery after surgery (ERAS) program and to patient blood management (PBM) program in the prospective observational multicenter iCral4 study [38]

also Chap. 18). The reappraisal of the iCral2 and iCral3 [28, 29] prospective multi-center studies on colorectal surgery in Italy showed that the incidence of infectious adverse events (a composite endpoint made up of surgical site, urinary tract, and pulmonary infections) significantly decreased from 7.7% in the first quartile (adherence rate ≤ 55%) to 3.0% in the fourth quartile (adherence rate > 85%) [30]. Compared to "older" perioperative care bundles such as ERAS, the PBM implementation process should be considered still in its infancy, and few data, if any, are available regarding sheer guidelines and related adherence rates. The only available, recently published, pre-post PBM implementation experience in colorectal cancer surgery from South Korea [31] clearly showed that notwithstanding a significant reduction of blood transfusions, the rate of infectious adverse events remained unaltered. However, as both intraoperative blood loss >600 mL and perioperative blood transfusions have been repeatedly identified as independent risk factors for SSIs [32–37], the role of a fully implemented PBM program in reducing infectious adverse events needs to be demonstrated through well-designed prospective studies. In the iCral4 study [38], a prospective multicenter observational study on elective colorectal surgery that has just closed accrual with more than 3500 patients enrolled in 60 Italian surgical centers, the median adherence rate to the ERAS program was beyond 70%, while that to the PBM program remained below 50% (Fig. 19.1). The road to full PBM implementation, therefore, is still long notwithstanding the existence of top-down directives from the Italian Ministry of Health and the Italian National Blood Center [39]. On the other hand, it is possible and advisable that recent bottom-up initiatives and recommendations from the involved scientific societies [40] will raise the compliance to PBM programs.

19.4 Conclusion

Both ERAS and PBM pathways are patient-centered, multidisciplinary, multifactorial, and evidence-based bundles of perioperative care measures designed to reduce the impact of major surgery on the patients' physiologic status. To date, the ERAS guideline recommendations include PBM measures limited to preoperative anemia screening and correction and intraoperative normothermia [41], while much remains to be implemented regarding postoperative anemia [19, 38]. At the same time, numerous international [42, 43] and national [44] guidelines have recently been made similarly available for infection prevention and control (IPC). Consequently, it appears logical that surgical scientific societies should move forward to the full implementation of these perioperative care bundles, monitoring adherence rates and results through a nationwide, continuous clinical audit. PBM, IPC, and ERAS should therefore be considered and benchmarked as a single bundle of evidence-based and patient-centered perioperative care measures.

Acknowledgements Some portions of this chapter have already been presented in authors' previously published papers [13, 19, 40].

References

1. Berríos-Torres SI, Umscheid CA, Bratzler DW, et al. Centers for Disease Control and Prevention guideline for the prevention of surgical site infection, 2017. JAMA Surg. 2017;152(8):784–91. Erratum in: JAMA Surg. 2017;152(8):803
2. Sanger PC, Hartzler A, Han SM, et al. Patient perspectives on post-discharge surgical site infections: towards a patient-centered mobile health solution. PLoS One. 2014;9(12):e114016.
3. World Health Organization. The urgent need to implement patient blood management: policy brief. WHO; 2021. https://www.who.int/publications/i/item/9789240035744. Accessed 16 Mar 2024
4. Sim YE, Wee HE, Ang AL, et al. Prevalence of preoperative anemia, abnormal mean corpuscular volume and red cell distribution width among surgical patients in Singapore, and their influence on one year mortality. PLoS One. 2017;12(8):e0182543.
5. Greenberg JA, Zwiep TM, Sadek J, et al. Clinical practice guideline: evidence, recommendations and algorithm for the preoperative optimization of anemia, hyperglycemia and smoking. Can J Surg. 2021;64(5):E491–509. Erratum in: Can J Surg. 2021;64(6):E619
6. Fowler AJ, Ahmad T, Phull MK, et al. Meta-analysis of the association between preoperative anaemia and mortality after surgery. Br J Surg. 2015;102(11):1314–24.
7. Beattie WS, Karkouti K, Wijeysundera DN, Tait G. Risk associated with preoperative anemia in noncardiac surgery: a single-center cohort study. Anesthesiology. 2009;110(3):574–81.
8. Muñoz M, Acheson AG, Auerbach M, et al. International consensus statement on the perioperative management of anaemia and iron deficiency. Anaesthesia. 2017;72(2):233–47.
9. Ponnusamy KE, Kim TJ, Khanuja HS. Perioperative blood transfusions in orthopaedic surgery. J Bone Joint Surg Am. 2014;96(21):1836–44.
10. Kumar A. Perioperative management of anemia: limits of blood transfusion and alternatives to it. Cleve Clin J Med. 2009;76(Suppl 4):S112–8.
11. Saleh A, Small T, Chandran Pillai AL, et al. Allogenic blood transfusion following total hip arthroplasty: results from the nationwide inpatient sample, 2000 to 2009. J Bone Joint Surg Am. 2014;96(18):e155.
12. Italian ColoRectal Anastomotic Leakage (iCral) Study Group. Risk factors for adverse events after elective colorectal surgery: beware of blood transfusions. Updat Surg. 2020;72(3):811–9.
13. Catarci M, Guadagni S, Masedu F, et al. Blood transfusions and adverse events after colorectal surgery: a propensity-score-matched analysis of a hen-egg issue. Diagnostics (Basel). 2023;13(5):952.

14. Opelz G, Sengar DP, Mickey MR, Terasaki PI. Effect of blood transfusions on subsequent kidney transplants. Transplant Proc. 1973;5(1):253–9.
15. Vamvakas EC, Blajchman MA. Transfusion-related immunomodulation (TRIM): an update. Blood Rev. 2007;21(6):327–48.
16. McSorley ST, Tham A, Dolan RD, et al. Perioperative blood transfusion is associated with postoperative systemic inflammatory response and poorer outcomes following surgery for colorectal cancer. Ann Surg Oncol. 2020;27(3):833–43.
17. Kapur R, Kim M, Rebetz J, et al. Gastrointestinal microbiota contributes to the development of murine transfusion-related acute lung injury. Blood Adv. 2018;2(13):1651–63.
18. D'Alessandro A, Zolla L. Proteomic analysis of red blood cells and the potential for the clinic: what have we learned so far? Expert Rev Proteomics. 2017;14(3):243–52.
19. Catarci M, Borghi F, Ficari F, Scatizzi M. Perioperative anemia and its implications. G Chir. 2022;42(1):e01.
20. Farmer SL, Trentino KM, Hofmann A, et al. A programmatic approach to patient blood management—reducing transfusions and improving patient outcomes. Open Anesthesiol J. 2015;9:6–16.
21. Roman MA, Abbasciano RG, Pathak S, et al. Patient blood management interventions do not lead to important clinical benefits or cost-effectiveness for major surgery: a network meta-analysis. Br J Anaesth. 2021;126(1):149–56.
22. Rohde JM, Dimcheff DE, Blumberg N, et al. Health care-associated infection after red blood cell transfusion: a systematic review and meta-analysis. JAMA. 2014;311(13):1317–26. Erratum in: JAMA. 2014;312(19):2045
23. Carson JL, Stanworth SJ, Dennis JA, et al. Transfusion thresholds for guiding red blood cell transfusion. Cochrane Database Syst Rev. 2021;12(12):CD002042.
24. Nelson G, Kiyang LN, Crumley ET, et al. Implementation of Enhanced Recovery After Surgery (ERAS) across a provincial healthcare system: the ERAS Alberta Colorectal Surgery experience. World J Surg. 2016;40(5):1092–103.
25. Ripollés-Melchor J, Ramírez-Rodríguez JM, Casans-Francés R, et al. Association between use of Enhanced Recovery After Surgery protocol and postoperative complications in colorectal surgery: the Postoperative Outcomes Within Enhanced Recovery After Surgery Protocol (POWER) study. JAMA Surg. 2019;154(8):725–36. Erratum in: JAMA Surg. 2022;157(5):460
26. Berian JR, Ban KA, Liu JB, et al. Adherence to enhanced recovery protocols in NSQIP and association with colectomy outcomes. Ann Surg. 2019;269(3):486–93.
27. Catarci M, Benedetti M, Maurizi A, et al. ERAS pathway in colorectal surgery: structured implementation program and high adherence for improved outcomes. Updat Surg. 2021;73(1):123–37.
28. Catarci M, Ruffo G, Viola MG, et al. ERAS program adherence-institutionalization, major morbidity and anastomotic leakage after elective colorectal surgery: the iCral2 multicenter prospective study. Surg Endosc. 2022;36(6):3965–84.
29. Italian ColoRectal Anastomotic Leakage (iCral) Study Group. Patient-reported outcomes, return to intended oncological therapy and enhanced recovery pathways after colorectal surgery: a prospective multicenter observational investigation by the Italian ColoRectal Anastomotic Leakage (iCral 3) study group. Ann Surg Open. 2023;4:e267.
30. Catarci M, Ruffo G, Viola MG, et al. High adherence to enhanced recovery pathway independently reduces major morbidity and mortality rates after colorectal surgery: a reappraisal of the iCral2 and iCral3 multicenter prospective studies. G Chir. 2023;43:e24.
31. Shin SH, Piozzi GN, Kwak JM, et al. Effect of a Patient Blood Management system on perioperative transfusion practice and short-term outcomes of colorectal cancer surgery. Blood Transfus. 2022;20(6):475–82.
32. Tang R, Chen HH, Wang YL, et al. Risk factors for surgical site infection after elective resection of the colon and rectum: a single-center prospective study of 2,809 consecutive patients. Ann Surg. 2001;234(2):181–9.
33. Bernard AC, Davenport DL, Chang PK, et al. Intraoperative transfusion of 1 U to 2 U packed red blood cells is associated with increased 30-day mortality, surgical-site infection, pneumonia, and sepsis in general surgery patients. J Am Coll Surg. 2009;208(5):931–7.

34. Campbell DA Jr, Henderson WG, Englesbe MJ, et al. Surgical site infection prevention: the importance of operative duration and blood transfusion—results of the first American College of Surgeons-National Surgical Quality Improvement Program Best Practices Initiative. J Am Coll Surg. 2008;207(6):810–20.
35. Glance LG, Dick AW, Mukamel DB, et al. Association between intraoperative blood transfusion and mortality and morbidity in patients undergoing noncardiac surgery. Anesthesiology. 2011;114(2):283–92.
36. Ejaz A, Schmidt C, Johnston FM, et al. Risk factors and prediction model for inpatient surgical site infection after major abdominal surgery. J Surg Res. 2017;217:153–9.
37. Mazzeffi M, Tanaka K, Galvagno S. Red blood cell transfusion and surgical site infection after colon resection surgery: a cohort study. Anesth Analg. 2017;125(4):1316–21.
38. Enhanced Recovery and Patient Blood Management in Colorectal Surgery: the Italian ColoRectal Anastomotic Leakage Study Group (iCral 4). ClinicalTrials.gov Id: NCT05227014. https://clinicaltrials.gov/ct2/show/NCT05227014. Accessed 16 Mar 2024
39. Ministero della Salute, Istituto Superiore di Sanità, Centro Nazionale Sangue. Linee Guida per il Programma di Patient Blood Management. LG CNS 05 Rev. 0 27/10/2016. https://www.centronazionalesangue.it/wp-content/uploads/2017/07/Linee-Guida-per-il-Programma-di-Patient-Blood-Management_0.pdf. Accessed 16 Mar 2024
40. Catarci M, Tritapepe L, Rondinelli MB, et al. Patient blood management in major digestive surgery: recommendations from the Italian multisociety (ACOI, SIAARTI, SIdEM, and SIMTI) modified Delphi consensus conference. G Chir. 2024;44(1):e41.
41. Mendez E, Puig G, Barquero M, et al. Enhanced recovery after surgery: a narrative review on patient blood management recommendations. Minerva Anestesiol. 2023;89(10):906–13.
42. World Health Organization. Global guidelines for the prevention of surgical site infection. 2nd ed. Geneva: WHO; 2018. https://www.who.int/publications/i/item/9789241550475. Accessed 16 Mar 2024
43. Sartelli M, Chichom-Mefire A, Labricciosa FM, et al. The management of intra-abdominal infections from a global perspective: 2017 WSES guidelines for management of intra-abdominal infections. World J Emerg Surg. 2017;12:29. Erratum in: World J Emerg Surg. 2017;12:36
44. Sartelli M, Cortese F, Scatizzi M, et al. ACOI Surgical Site Infections Management Academy (ACOISSIMA): recommendations on the prevention of surgical site infections. G Chir. 2022;42(2):e12.

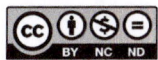

Financial Impact of Surgical Site Infections in Italy

20

Francesco Saverio Mennini, Paolo Sciattella, and Gabriele Sganga

20.1 Introduction

Surgical site infections not only affect patients' health and quality of life, but they also generate significant costs for healthcare services and the National Health Service (NHS), as they can impact the length of hospital stay and the need for additional therapies and treatments [1]. The objective of this chapter is to provide an estimate of the financial impact of surgical site infections in Italy using national real-world data.

20.2 Data Source and Methods

The analysis was conducted using the hospital discharge records provided by the Italian Ministry of Health containing information on admissions in public and private hospitals nationwide for the 2015–2021 period [2, 3].

First, the volume of admissions for surgical diagnosis-related groups (DRGs) and the proportion of surgical site infections were described. Surgical site infections

Supplementary Information The online version contains supplementary material available at https://doi.org/10.1007/978-3-031-60462-1_20.

F. S. Mennini (✉) · P. Sciattella
Economic Evaluation and HTA (EEHTA), Centre for Economics and International Studies,
Faculty of Economics, Tor Vergata University, Rome, Italy
e-mail: f.mennini@uniroma2.it; paolo.sciattella@uniroma2.it

G. Sganga
Emergency and Trauma Surgery Unit, Fondazione Policlinico
Universitario A. Gemelli IRCCS, Università Cattolica del Sacro Cuore, Rome, Italy
e-mail: gabriele.sganga@unicatt.it

© The Author(s) 2025
S. Bartoli et al. (eds.), *Infections in Surgery*, Updates in Surgery,
https://doi.org/10.1007/978-3-031-60462-1_20

were identified by selecting all acute hospitalizations occurring as regular admissions for "Infected postoperative seroma" (ICD-9 CM code 998.51) and/or "Other postoperative infections" (ICD-9 CM code 998.59).

Subsequently, an analysis focusing on the occurrence of postoperative infections following surgery was performed for the following six diseases:

- diverticulitis
- appendicitis
- cholecystitis
- cholelithiasis
- hernia
- ventral hernia.

Specifically, for each disease and related surgery, the incidence of postoperative infections was estimated, along with the resulting impact in terms of length of hospital stay and NHS expenditure. The surgeries of interest were identified by sorting hospital admissions based on information on the main diagnosis and main surgery (see the online Supplementary material of this chapter). Specifically, for each of the six diseases being examined, the ICD-9 CM diagnosis codes were used to identify the disease, while the ICD-9 CM procedure codes identify the related surgery.

The selected hospital stays were classified as "admissions with infection" (cases) and "admissions without infections" (controls), based on the presence/absence of the diagnosis of "Postoperative infected seroma" or "Other postoperative infection."

The increase in the length of hospital stay due to infections was estimated for each disease, comparing the average hospital stay with or without postoperative infections.

Similarly, the financial impact of surgical site infections was estimated comparing the economic value of hospital admissions with or without infections.

The theoretical valuation of hospital admissions was estimated based on the assumption that each admission would be paid according to the national tariff (established by the Ministry of Health) [4]. Therefore, the reported values do not correspond to the costs actually incurred for hospital services, but to the value of the payments borne by NHS for hospital services.

20.3   Results

In the period being analyzed 893,000 surgeries were selected, of which 38.3% are referred to cholecystitis, 19% to cholelithiasis, 15% to hernias and 13.7% to appendicitis.

The average occurrence of postoperative infections was 0.23%, ranging from 0.07% for hernia surgery and 1.35% for surgery of diverticulitis (Table 20.1).

The average length of hospital stay for the surgeries considered, in the absence of infections, was 5.1 days, ranging from 3.5 days in hospital for hernias and 13 days for diverticulitis. In the case of postoperative infection, the average length of

Table 20.1 Surgeries per disease and postoperative infections, Italy 2015–2021

Type of surgery	Hospital admissions	
	Without infection	With infections
Appendicitis	121,907 *(99.58%)*	513 *(0.42%)*
Cholelithiasis	170,519 *(99.92%)*	137 *(0.08%)*
Cholecystitis	342,899 *(99.83%)*	587 *(0.17%)*
Diverticulitis	30,522 *(98.63%)*	419 *(1.37%)*
Hernia	134,386 *(99.93%)*	94 *(0.07%)*
Ventral hernia	93,739 *(99.71%)*	271 *(0.29%)*
Total	**893,972** *(99.77%)*	**2021** *(0.23%)*

Source: Authors' analysis of hospital discharge data

Table 20.2 Average hospital stay per disease without and with postoperative infections, Italy 2015–2021

Type of surgery	Average hospital stay		Increase of length of stay attributable to postoperative infection
	Without infection	With infections	
Appendicitis	4.7	12.6	7.9
Cholelithiasis	4.1	21.3	17.2
Cholecystitis	5.6	19.0	13.4
Diverticulitis	13.3	22.7	9.3
Hernia	3.5	10.7	7.3
Ventral hernia	5.3	20.2	14.9
Total	**5.1**	**18.1**	**13.0**

Source: Authors' analysis of hospital discharge data

hospital stay increased to 18.1, ranging from 10.7 for hernia to 22.7 for diverticulitis. Therefore, the average increase in the length of hospital stay attributable to postoperative infections was around 13 days, up to a maximum of 17 days observed in hospital stays for surgery of ventral hernia (Table 20.2).

The estimate of the average financial impact of postoperative infections was calculated considering the theoretical value of the payments based on DRG tariffs.

The occurrence of postoperative infections leds to an average increase in the expenditure borne by the Italian NHS of €4424 per single hospital admission. Indeed, in the absence of infections, the expenditure was €3343, while it increased to €7768 if infections occurred.

The highest financial impact was recorded for cholelithiasis-related surgeries (+ €4174) and for ventral hernia (+ €3758) (Table 20.3).

Considering that the theoretical value of hospital admission does not change as a function of the length of stay, assuming it remains within the DRG-specific threshold value, the financial impact of infections arising during hospitalization was also

Table 20.3 Average expenditure per hospital admission per disease without and with postoperative infections, Italy 2015–2021

Type of surgery	Hospital admissions expenditure (€)		Increase of expenditure (€) attributable to postoperative infection
	Without infection	With infections	
Appendicitis	3176	5550	2374
Cholelithiasis	3344	7518	4174
Cholecystitis	3617	7128	3511
Diverticulitis	10,616	13,113	2497
Hernia	1593	4180	2587
Ventral hernia	2697	6455	3758
Total	**3343**	**7768**	**4424**

Source: Authors' analysis of hospital discharge data

Table 20.4 Financial impact of postoperative infections, Italy 2015–2021

Type of surgery	Total financial impact (€) attributable to postoperative infections	%
Appendicitis	3,330,148	17.7
Cholelithiasis	1,934,046	10.3
Cholecystitis	6,465,030	34.4
Diverticulitis	3,215,941	17.1
Hernia	559,861	3.0
Ventral hernia	3,306,776	17.6
Total	**18,811,802**	**100.0**

Source: Authors' analysis of hospital discharge data

calculated by valuing the number of additional hospital days attributable to infections. The valuation was calculated considering the average cost of a day of hospital stay at national level reported in the "green book" on public spending issued by the Italian Ministry of Economy and Finance [5], updated to 2018 (median year of the period under study) and equal to €821.

The total financial impact attributable to postoperative infections, over the period being analyzed, was €18.8 million (Table 20.4).

20.4 Conclusion

The analysis of postoperative infections following surgeries of the six diseases considered showed a major impact in terms of length of hospital stay and expenditure borne by the Italian NHS. Indeed, based on about 800,000 surgeries considered, postoperative infections occurred in 23 cases per 10,000, resulting in an average increase of 13 days in the length of hospital stay and an increase of €4242 in the expenditure per hospital stay.

Valuing the increase in hospital stay with the average cost per hospital day, the total impact of the postoperative infections identified was €18.8 million.

The increase in length of hospital stay due to the occurrence of infections generates an increase in costs for hospital care. In addition, it entails indirect costs related to the loss of productivity of working-age patients and any caregivers.

It should also be noted that the results of this analysis should be considered partial, as they do not take into account the impact of postoperative infections in terms of social security costs. Moreover, we should take into account the huge impact of non-medical costs borne by the public healthcare system arising from civil litigation due to patient claims following hospital infections.

References

1. The European House—Ambrosetti. Meridiano Sanità Report 2022, 17th Edition. https://acad-min.ambrosetti.eu/dompdf/crea_wmark.php?doc=L2F0dGFjaG1lbnRzL3BkZi9yYXBwb3J0 by1tZXJpZGlhbm8tc2FuaXRhLTE3LTIwMjItMjAyMjExMTAxNi5wZGY%3D&id=16841 &muid=corporate. Accessed 16 Mar 2024.
2. Ministero della Salute. Il flusso informativo SDO, 4 dicembre 2008 (ultimo aggiornamento 12 febbraio 2024) [Italian Ministry of Health. Data flow of hospital discharge records, 4 December 2008. Last update 12 February 2024. https://www.salute.gov.it/portale/temi/p2_6.jsp?lingua=it aliano&id=1232&area=ricoveriOspedalieri&menu=rilevazione. Accessed 16 Mar 2024
3. Ministero della Salute. Rapporti annuali sull'attività di ricovero ospedaliero, 8 febbraio 2024 [Italian Ministry of Health. Annual reports on hospitalization, 8 February 2024]. https://www.salute.gov.it/portale/temi/p2_6.jsp?lingua=italiano&id=1237&area=ricoveriOspedalieri&men u=vuotolink. Accessed 16 Mar 2024
4. Ministero della Salute. Decreto 21 dicembre 2012: Aggiornamento degli importi delle tariffe e dei diritti per le prestazioni rese a richiesta ed a utilità dei soggetti interessati [Italian Ministry of Health. Decree 21 December 2012: Update of tariffs and fees for the services rendered upon request of and for the benefit of interested parties]. https://www.gazzettaufficiale.it/atto/serie_generale/caricaDettaglioAtto/originario?atto.dataPubblicazioneGazzetta=2013-03-15& atto.codiceRedazionale=13A02275&elenco30giorni=true. Accessed 16 Mar 2024
5. Ministero dell'Economia e delle Finanze—Commissione Tecnica per la Finanza Pubblica. Libro verde sulla spesa pubblica, 6 settembre 2007 [Ministry of Economy and Finance—Technical Commission on Public Finance. Green book on public spending, 6 September 2007]. https://www.mef.gov.it/ministero/commissioni/ctfp/documenti/Libro_verde_spesa_pubblica. pdf. Accessed 16 Mar 2024

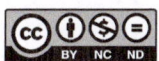

The Legal Impact of Infections in Surgery Under Italian Law

21

Dalila Ranalletta

The term "healthcare-associated infections" (HAIs) has long replaced earlier terms such as "nosocomial infections" and "hospital infections", as the evidence shows that infections may occur within any care setting. Among the several existing scientific and lay definitions of HAIs, the Italian Ministry of Health has adopted the following:

> Healthcare-associated infections (HAIs) are acquired infections that represent the most frequent and severe complication of health care and can occur within any care setting, including acute care facilities, day-hospital/day-surgery facilities, long-term care facilities, outpatient clinics, home care services and community residential facilities. HAIs include infections transmitted from sources outside the body (exogenous), from person to person or via health professionals and the healthcare environment, and infections caused by bacteria found inside the body (endogenous) [1].

HAIs account for a particularly significant number of adverse events, such as to cause constant concern within the scientific community, both because they represent an extremely complex public health issue and because they entail a considerable social and economic burden. The problem has therefore been addressed by issuing guidelines and recommendations (both national and international) which, while undoubtedly providing useful tools for the prevention and control of HAIs, have not been able to prevent the adoption of widely differing policies at the regional and local level.

In contrast to the scientific ferment on the subject, the possibility of medical liability arising from a HAI has, over the years, brought to light the high level of complexity involved in ascertaining the causal links. In this regard, it should first be underlined that there is consensus on the need to distinguish between:

D. Ranalletta (✉)
Forensic Medicine Unit, ASL Roma 1, Rome, Italy
e-mail: dalila.ranalletta@libero.it

© The Author(s) 2025
S. Bartoli et al. (eds.), *Infections in Surgery*, Updates in Surgery,
https://doi.org/10.1007/978-3-031-60462-1_21

- *the legal causal link*: this is the link that "must be ascertained between the specific conduct and a specific event in order for 'structural' liability (*haftungsbegründenden Kausalität*) to arise" [2];
- *the material causal link*: that is, the one which, "by linking the event to the specific damage/harm, enables identification of the individual resulting harms, with the main aim of drawing the boundaries of an (already ascertained) compensatory liability (*haftungsausfüllenden Kausalität*)" [2].

Generally speaking, a person may be held liable for a tort or for a crime if a specific event has occurred as a result of his/her conduct. This direct connection is the *causal link*. If the conduct (an act or omission) is held to be reprehensible, however, it will first be necessary to establish the probability that the given conduct is or is not the cause of the event. In this respect, there is a considerable difference in the principles governing ascertainment of the causal link: in *criminal liability* the "beyond reasonable doubt" principle applies, whereas in *civil liability* the "more likely than not" principle applies. In practice, however, the degree of probability required within civil law proceedings is much lower than that found in criminal law proceedings.

Medicolegal (and jurisprudential) considerations in assessing a causal link must necessarily be based on a discipline-specific methodological approach, in that the existence of a causal link between the given conduct and the event must be investigated according to unavoidable criteria. In particular, it should be assessed whether any omission (in terms of prevention) occurred that is intrinsically capable of causing harm or whether the event would have occurred in any case irrespective of the conduct, to then apply different considerations depending on whether the case falls within the remit of criminal law or civil law.

From a medicolegal viewpoint, the difficulty in ascertaining the material causal link lies mainly in the vast array of factors generating the infection, but a further element of complexity stems from the need to provide the judge with the indispensable technical elements required to enable a fair and shareable assessment. Especially important among these elements (which are indeed numerous) is the identification of the rule of conduct to be adopted in cases similar to the one under examination and the possible demonstrable and documentable deviation from such rule.

The court-appointed medical expert (in Italian law, *consulente tecnico d'ufficio*, or CTU), having established by means of clinical investigations that the infection can be traced back to the healthcare facility, must first try to ascertain whether the infection was unavoidable (and therefore not preventable) or whether, on the contrary, it could have been effectively avoided by adopting all the precautions reported in the scientific literature (as well as in the guidelines, best practices and recommendations). In other words, the expert must first ascertain whether the infection is due to a circumstance that cannot be attributed directly to the healthcare facility or whether the conduct of the facility's healthcare staff presents profiles of fault/negligence that may be causally linked to the infection. It should also be recalled that the concept of "complication", which for many years was widely used by court-appointed medical experts, can no longer be invoked, as it is now a constant and undisputed assumption in jurisprudence that the clinical concept of complication is alien to the legal concept. This is well explained by several passages of the motivations of a 2015 ruling of the Court of Cassation (the Italian highest appellate court):

> With the term 'complication', clinical medicine and forensic medicine usually designate a harmful event arising in the course of a patient's treatment, which, although theoretically predictable, would be impossible to avoid. This concept is pointless in the legal sphere. Indeed, whenever a patient's condition worsens during or after completion of a surgical operation, there are two possibilities: either such worsening was predictable and avoidable, in which case it must be ascribed to the doctor's fault, notwithstanding the fact that clinical statistics theoretically classify it as a 'complication', or such worsening was not predictable or was not avoidable, in which case it constitutes an 'non-attributable cause', [...] irrespective of the fact that clinical statistics do not theoretically classify it as a 'complication' [3].

In the event that the causal link between an infection and the provision of specific healthcare services is established, the healthcare facility will need to rebut the "presumption" of liability by providing proof of its innocence with regard to the hypothesis of not having complied with the rules of HAI prevention and management. For a considerable period of time, the question was what proof the healthcare facility should give other than the obvious provision of documentation of all internal procedures aimed at preventing and managing infections. This, in fact, proved to be effective in demonstrating that the healthcare facility had correctly implemented all the appropriate prevention measures to combat hospital infections; basically, with the easily imaginable differences between the various settings, these prevention measures include actions concerning sterilization and ventilation systems, constant monitoring of staff, patient and environmental hygiene, an appropriate information flow enabling the identification and quantification of infections in the various facilities, the training of the staff involved in patient care and especially in the critical areas of intensive care and surgery. However, over time such documentation proved to be totally insufficient to discharge the burden of proof falling to the healthcare facility, since recent rulings have almost constantly tended to demand that the healthcare facility provide exonerating proof (a requirement defined "diabolical" by some), i.e., the facility has to demonstrate that the documented protocols were actually applied.

In practice, recent years have seen a new trend in case law (even in the absence of any formal and explicit recognition to this effect) to configure hypotheses of liability that some have defined as a 'true hypothesis of strict liability' (i.e., that liability placed on the subject without any blame or malice being attributed to them, sanctioned by Article 42 of the Italian Penal Code [4]), thus solving the issue of ascertaining the fault of the healthcare facility with arguments that can be summarized essentially as follows:

– a hospital must be an aseptic place;
– the patient contracted the infection inside the hospital, hence asepsis was not guaranteed;
– ergo, the failure to ensure perfect asepsis was the fault of the healthcare professionals.

And even if the healthcare facility should succeed in proving that it had always sanitized the staff and the operating areas according to precise protocols, it will receive the answer that, since the infection occurred despite its action, the disinfection procedures must not have been performed correctly. This is an extreme application of the *res ipsa loquitur* principle, in the light of which the plaintiff rarely loses at the end of the trial.

Therefore, the absence of documentation clearly demonstrating how the healthcare facility effectively implemented the preventive procedures and how such procedures were implemented by the healthcare staff means that the infection is deemed to be causally related to organizational deficiencies of the healthcare facility and/or failures of the healthcare personnel. Moreover, the circumstance that the patient, due to his/her intrinsic characteristics (age, pre-existing conditions), was particularly at risk of developing a nosocomial infection is of no relevance: on the contrary, the presence of risk factors represents a further reason for the healthcare facility to pay greater attention to prevention measures.

Coming to the rescue of healthcare facilities, in the light of this trend and the consequent almost constant succumbing of healthcare facilities in proceedings concerning compensation for damages referring to hospital infections, the Court of Cassation intervened in 2023 with a clarifying ruling [5]. With reference to nosocomial infections, the Court first of all specified in detail the nature of the burden of proof that falls to the healthcare facility and/or doctor in order to be exempted from liability, definitively establishing that this is not a form of objective liability.

Referring to previous rulings [6, 7] rendered by the same, the Court preliminarily reiterated the following principles:

> It falls to the patient to prove the causal link between the worsening of his/her pathological condition (or the onset of new pathological conditions) and the conduct of the healthcare professional, while it falls to the healthcare facility to prove that it has performed the service correctly or to prove the unpredictable and unavoidable cause of the impossibility of performing such service correctly. With special reference to nosocomial infections, it falls to the healthcare facility to prove: 1) that the facility has adopted all the precautionary measures prescribed by the regulations in force and under the *leges artis*, in order to prevent the onset of infectious diseases; 2) that the facility and its staff have applied the infection prevention protocols in the specific case in question; thus proving that the specific case does not entail a hypothesis of strict liability [5].

That being stated, the ruling lists the items of a check list detailing the information the healthcare facilities should attach and demonstrate in order to be granted exemption from liability, and specifying the documentation to be produced in court [5]:

(a) The provision of protocols for disinfection, disinfestation and sterilization of environments and materials;
(b) The procedure in place for collecting, washing and disinfecting linen;
(c) The procedures in place for solid waste and sewage disposal;
(d) The technical features of the catering service and the means of distributing food and beverages;
(e) The procedures in place for preparing, storing and using disinfectants;

(f) Air quality and air conditioning systems;
(g) The activation of a video surveillance and notification system;
(h) The indication of criteria for controlling and limiting visitor access;
(i) Staff injury and illness control procedures and vaccination prophylaxis;
(j) An indication of the staff-to-inpatient ratio;
(k) Surveillance based on microbiological laboratory data;
(l) The preparation of reports by the heads of the departments to be communicated to the medical directorates in order to monitor pathogenic sentinel germs;
(m) The scheduling of the actual execution of risk prevention activities.

Within the same ruling, the Court of Cassation also deals with another aspect, pertaining to the role of the personnel employed at the facility, from the top management position down to the operational units, on which the court-appointed experts should also be called upon to express an opinion regarding liability, clearly with the aim of identifying the person responsible for the infection, an aspect that pertains more to the possible action for compensation of the healthcare facility or the Corte dei Conti (Italian Court of Auditors).

In particular, the Court of Cassation specifies in detail which subjective obligations are incumbent on each position within the hospital organization [5]:

– The hospital director general has the obligation to set out the precautionary rules to be implemented and the power/duty to supervise and check their implementation (periodic meetings/visits), as also done by the Infection Control Committee;
– The medical director is required to implement such rules, to arrange the necessary hygiene and technical-sanitary procedures and to monitor the implementation of the rules (Article 5 of Presidential Decree 128/1969 [8]: obligation to draw up protocols for sterilization and environmental sanitation, management of medical records, supervision of informed consent);
– The head of department, who is the final executor of both protocols and guidelines, is required to cooperate with the specialists (microbiologist, infectiologist, epidemiologist, hygienist), and is liable for failure to collect accurate information on the initiatives taken by other physicians or for failure to report possible shortcomings to those in charge.

It can therefore be seen how the 2023 ruling of the Court of Cassation introduced important innovations, i.e., the "new guidelines" that will necessarily have to be adopted, although it still remains to be seen what their practical and systemic implications will be.

Therefore, the Court established important rules within the judicial compensation procedures. In particular, it definitively established that, in response to a claim for damages due to the consequences suffered for having contracted a healthcare-related infection, the healthcare facility will have to prove not only that it has arranged a series of specific activities aimed at preventing the risk of infection, but it will also have to provide proof that it has implemented them.

The analytical structure of the documentation to be prepared and provided to discharge the burden of proof entails unquestionable difficulties for the healthcare facilities (and for top management and non-executive managers) in preparing and collecting all the documentation listed. However, it is equally beyond doubt that these are valuable indications that help to prepare the documentation to be attached in court to demonstrate that they have concretely adopted all the measures useful for the prevention and management of the risk of infection. Lastly, the Court of Cassation also intervened on the duties of the court-appointed experts in order for them to correctly assess the causal relationship between the infection and the harm. Specifically, the Court postulates:

> They will investigate both general and specific causality, on the one hand excluding, if necessary, the sufficiency of general recommendations regarding the prevention of clinical risk and, on the other, avoiding a 'mechanical' implementation of the *post hoc-propter hoc* criterion, and thus examining the clinical history of the patient, the nature and quality of the protocols, the characteristics of the specific microorganism and the mapping of the microbial flora present within the individual wards: the court-appointed expert should therefore be asked a composite question, specifically addressed to ascertaining the etiological relationship between the infection and the hospital stay in relation to situations such as the following:
>
> (a) lack of or insufficient general directives on prevention (responsibility of the director general and medical director and the Infection Control Committee);
> (b) failure to comply with adequate and efficiently publicized directives (liability of the head of department and the department healthcare staff), failure to provide information on the possible inadequacy of the facility due to unavailability of essential instruments [...], and hospitalizations not supported by any diagnostic and therapeutic need and associated with inappropriate treatment. [5]

In practical terms, what the court requires in cases of HAI is that the facility provide not only proof of the existence of the procedures, but also proof that such procedures have been widely implemented and adhered to in the specific case under examination, while also taking into account the liability attributable to poor organization and/or faulty operation of equipment, which might have been avoided by means of targeted company investments. All this, despite the painful awareness that, irrespective of the greatest attention being paid to prevention and management measures, healthcare-related infections continue to account for a significant proportion of the statistics concerning adverse healthcare outcomes.

References

1. Ministero della Salute. Infezioni correlate all'assistenza: cosa sono e cosa fare (aggiornamento 8 settembre 2022) [Italian Ministry of Health. Healthcare-associated infections: what they are and what to do (updated 8 September 2022)]. The online Supplementary material of this chapter. https://www.salute.gov.it/portale/malattieInfettive/dettaglioContenutiMalattieInfettive.jsp?lingua=italiano&id=648&area=Malattie%20infettive&menu=icain.
2. Corte di Cassazione, Sezione III Civile, Sentenza 16 ottobre 2007, n. 21619 [Italian Court of Cassation, Civil Section III, Ruling 16 October 2007, n. 21619].

3. Corte di Cassazione, Sezione III Civile, Sentenza 30 giugno 2015, n. 13328 [Italian Court of Cassation, Civil Section III, Ruling 30 June 2015, n. 13328].
4. Codice Penale, Art. 42—Responsabilità per dolo o per colpa o per delitto preterintenzionale. Responsabilità obiettiva [Italian Penal Code, Art. 42—Liability for intent or negligence or unpremeditated crime. Objective liability].
5. Corte di Cassazione, Sezione III Civile, Sentenza 3 marzo 2023, n. 6386 [Italian Court of Cassation, Civil Section III, Ruling 3 March 2023, n. 6386].
6. Corte di Cassazione, Sezione III Civile, Sentenza 23 febbraio 2021, n. 4864 [Italian Court of Cassation, Civil Section III, Ruling 23 February 2021, n. 4864].
7. Corte di Cassazione, Sezione III Civile, Sentenza 15 giugno 2020, n.11599 [Italian Court of Cassation, Civil Section III, Ruling 15 June 2020, n.11599].
8. Decreto del Presidente della Repubblica 27 marzo 1969, n. 128—Ordinamento interno dei servizi ospedalieri [Decree of the President of the Republic, 27 March 1969, n.128—Internal organization of hospital services].

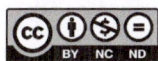

The Strategic Role of Health Technology Assessment Within the Surgical Infection Setting

22

Emanuela Foglia, Lucrezia Ferrario,
and Elisabetta Garagiola

22.1 Relevance of Technological Governance and the Role of Health Technology Assessment

In an era characterized by rapid advancements in medical science and technology, by an increasingly aging population, growing frailty and chronic illnesses, the healthcare landscape faces a multifaceted set of challenges, leading to a significant increase in healthcare expenditure.

Another driver impacting healthcare costs is the development of innovative healthcare technologies [1], represented not only by drugs, medical devices or equipment used in clinical practice, but also by medical, surgical, and laboratory procedures to attain desired patient outcomes [2]. All healthcare technologies can be assessed not only from the point of view of the National Health System (NHS) (institutional level), but also from the perspectives of both the hospital (meso level) and the individual clinical practice (micro level), with respect to the impact they may have on the different organizational settings in terms of patient outcomes, healthcare costs and societal well-being.

However, a question is still open: "How to effectively evaluate healthcare technologies? Which tools are best suited for defining the validity and sustainability of a healthcare intervention?"

Traditionally, healthcare decision-making processes have been dominated by two primary criteria: efficacy and cost (considering both the NHS and the hospital perspective).

In Italy, the control mechanisms introduced by legislation to monitor and regulate healthcare expenditure have shown a gradual decline in effectiveness over time: attention was focused on efficiency and productivity measures rather than on the

E. Foglia (✉) · L. Ferrario · E. Garagiola
Healthcare Data Science LAB—HD LAB, LIUC-Cattaneo University,
Castellanza (Varese), Italy
e-mail: efoglia@liuc.it; lferrario@liuc.it; egaragiola@liuc.it

© The Author(s) 2025
S. Bartoli et al. (eds.), *Infections in Surgery*, Updates in Surgery,
https://doi.org/10.1007/978-3-031-60462-1_22

relations between available resources and population health outcomes. This called for the adoption of alternative tools, particularly those inherent to clinical governance, aimed at enhancing "the quality of services and preserving high standards of care, fostering an environment conducive to healthcare excellence" [3].

Among all the clinical governance tools, Health Technology Assessment (HTA) has emerged as a strategic component for supporting decisions regarding appropriateness and quality in resource utilization, and has proved to be a systematic and multidisciplinary process that evaluates the clinical effectiveness, safety, cost-effectiveness, societal and organizational impact of the development, introduction, and dissemination of technologies [4].

The main objective of HTA is to provide a comprehensive and evidence-based approach to evaluating health technologies, helping healthcare systems make informed decisions that lead to better patient care, efficient resource allocation and improved health outcomes, guiding the integration and governance of technologies in healthcare systems.

HTA can be used throughout the entire technology's life cycle evaluating its ongoing impact and appropriateness. It can be applied during the early stages of technology development to assess the potential benefits, costs, and risks of a new technology, helping to make informed decisions about whether to proceed with further development or research [4]. HTA can be used to monitor the safety and effectiveness of a technology after its real-life introduction, providing ongoing evaluation of its real-world performance and identifying any unexpected or long-term effects [5]. Moreover, HTA can continually assess the cost-effectiveness of the technology, considering not only the initial acquisition costs but also the long-term economic impact, such as cost savings or increased costs due to complications.

Based on these premises, HTA can be applied to any healthcare technologies, including also those impacting the field of surgical site infections (SSIs), to evaluate new interventions that are constantly being developed [6] and allow decision-makers to prioritize resources based on the potential return on investment, while aligning clinical practice with patient-centered care [7].

22.2 Focus on the Dimensions of Health Technology Assessment

The European Network of Health Technology Assessment (EUnetHTA) has suggested a standardized technique to evaluate any healthcare technology. This model, called the EUnetHTA Corel Model, proposes the analysis of nine "dimensions" (or "domains"): health problem and current use of technology; description and technical characteristics; safety; clinical efficacy; economic and financial impact; equity analysis; organizational aspects; ethical and social aspects; legal aspects (Table 22.1).

Different data sources are usually employed to assess the HTA dimensions: (1) scientific evidence available in the literature, in particular for assessment of the clinical domains (efficacy and safety) and for identifying the target population (e.g., number of patients with SSI that may be eligible for an innovative technology); (2)

Table 22.1 The main Health Technology Assessment dimensions, within their specific rationale

Dimension	Rationale of the dimension
Health problem and current use of technology	A thorough description of the pathology is provided in this section, including prevalence and incidence data that should refer to the local or national context in which the decision will be taken. To further comprehend the need for technological use, this dimension also aims to define the eligible target population that would benefit from the use of innovative technology
Description and technical characteristics	This domain aims at identifying the technical indicators related to the new technology and the alternatives. As a result, it identifies the primary distinctions between technologies, describing their advantages and disadvantages from a strictly technical and scientific point of view
Safety	This dimension contains details about the safety profile of the technologies under investigation, such as potential side effects or complications from their use that could have a negative impact on both effectiveness and outcomes as well as the cost of the hospital activities needed to address and manage such side effects. Data would usually derive from literature evidence available on the topic and, whenever possible, from local registries or hospital databases
Clinical efficacy	This domain enables the definition of "clinical effectiveness" and the identification of benefits associated with the application of the innovative technology. It is important to assess the clinical efficacy and effectiveness of surgical infection interventions, including surgical procedures, antimicrobial agents, and infection prevention strategies. This dimension would thus include the assessment of the efficacy of infection control and prevention strategies, such as preoperative antibiotics, aseptic techniques, and protocols for reducing surgical site infections. Data would usually derive from literature evidence available on the topic and, whenever possible, from local registries or hospital databases
Economic impact	This dimension defines the costs associated with the adoption of the innovative technology, with respect to the standard of care, assuming both the hospital and/or the National Healthcare Service perspectives. It is important to examine the utilization of healthcare resources, such as hospital length of stay, readmission rates, and the need for additional surgeries or treatments. After having identified all the economic resources absorbed for the management of a patient, the economic impact would include both a cost-effectiveness analysis (identifying the technology with the best trade-off between expenses incurred and results realized) and a budget impact analysis (defining the financial sustainability of the technology, considering the budget holder perspective)
Equity analysis	This aspect defines the technologies' accessibility and availability within the local context of reference, as well as identifying any patient groups that may be adversely affected by the introduction of new technologies. The evaluation of this domain would also result in the definition of a possible change to local healthcare access, which would improve hospital waiting lists
Organizational aspects	This dimension aims at assessing the investments or disinvestments that the new technology may create by evaluating the impact of the technology within the considered unit of analysis (operating unit, health facility, etc.). A thorough assessment of the workforce, training, and structural modifications is needed: As such the organizational costs are determined. In addition, a qualitative method should be used to assess this domain, gathering the opinions of healthcare practitioners, to define their intention to use the innovative technology
Ethical and social aspects	This aspect would define not only patient-reported experiences and outcomes (from a qualitative perspective), but also quantify the patients' productivity loss due to the management of any surgical infection
Legal aspects	This domain would assess the regulatory and policy implications of the management of surgical infection interventions, including compliance with healthcare regulations and the potential need for policy changes to improve patient outcomes

real-life data useful for applying the health economics tools to be used to assess the quantitative economic and organizational domains; (3) stakeholders' opinions and points of view.

The integration of various data sources and different perspectives will bring together experts from numerous disciplines, such as medicine, health economics, health policy, ethics, and social sciences, to ensure a comprehensive evaluation of the technology's benefits, risks, costs, and broader implications, also giving insights into the main drivers that may enhance the acceptance and intention-to-use of any technologies, thus structuring an informed decision-making process.

22.3   Health Technology Assessment and Surgical Site Infections

SSIs increase the risk of postoperative mortality and morbidity, which extends length of hospital stay (LOS), and necessitates additional SSI-related surgical procedures, with an impact on health expenditure [8, 9]. Given the importance of SSIs, innovative technologies may play a key role in their prevention and management in terms of both new hospital procedures and protocols and implementation of new medical devices requiring the adoption of HTA techniques.

Despite the possible higher acquisition cost, the adoption of innovative technologies could help reduce costs incurred in the event of a complication, supporting the goal to achieve better patient outcomes throughout the surgical site healing continuum. Thus, SSI surveillance is crucial issue for the healthcare system and access to the best available therapy or strategy to control and reduce SSI incidence is essential. HTA should address this urgency by evaluating various interventions within specific target patient populations (e.g., pediatric, geriatric, immunocompromised) that may have different health needs.

An Italian study [10] investigated the absorption of economic resources for the management of patients developing or not developing SSI after surgery, by considering all general, cardiac, obstetric-gynecologic, and orthopedic surgical procedures conducted within a medium-size Italian hospital over a 12-month period. The medical management of a complication would generate a significant increase in hospital costs, especially as a result of increased LOS (+64%) and the need to perform additional operations to resolve the complications (+42%). However, the authors reported that the implementation of a specific portable device for negative pressure wound therapy (NPWT), able to reduce the risk of SSI (from 50% for obstetric-gynecologic surgery [11] to 93% for cardiac surgery [12]) would lead to an overall reduction in hospital costs of −0.69% and organizational savings due to shorter LOS equal to −1.10%, which could be reinvested to allow additional surgical procedures. Although the portable device for NPWT would have a higher acquisition cost than standard antibiotic prophylaxis, hospitals could ensure that patients experience a more effective pathway, leading to improved performance and patient satisfaction, and generating a positive impact that, based on an HTA approach, affects not only the economic dimension but also the organizational sphere, with important benefits in terms of access to care, and patients' quality of life.

Focusing on the prevention of surgical infections, reducing the risk of infectious complications has been linked to maintaining appropriate blood flow and tissue oxygenation, revealing the importance of maintaining tissue temperature. On the contrary, inadvertent perioperative hypothermia (IPH) is related to clinically significant negative outcomes, including increased bleeding, cerebral ischemia episodes, SSI, delayed wound healing, and hemorrhagic events due to coagulation inhibition [13]. This condition could be prevented through central temperature monitoring and patient warming in all perioperative phases [14]; additionally, "forced-air warming (FAW) appears to have a beneficial effect in terms of a lower rate of SSIs compared with no active warming system" [15]. Given the proven efficacy and safety profiles of such methods, a recent study was conducted to understand, based on an HTA approach, the economic and organizational impact of the introduction of FAW into clinical practice, and to assess both the patients' perspective and the healthcare professionals' perceptions on the technology [16]. From an economic viewpoint, FAW adoption may lead to savings of 16% per patient, thus enabling a higher efficacy level while optimizing the patient's pathway compared to no device being used. From a social and organizational viewpoint, the use of FAW technology was related to significant advantages: the social cost was reduced by 30% and the number of overall hospital days was reduced by between 15% and 26%. Moreover, the qualitative analyses of the perceptions of the healthcare professionals directly involved in the process confirmed that FAW technology was widely preferred. Therefore, based on an HTA analysis, the authors were able to conclude that FAW adoption can significantly improve patient outcomes and avoid IPH, demonstrating its strategic relevance.

In an attempt to prevent and/or decrease SSIs, the standard of care is represented by traditional dressing or advanced wound care. However, traditional wound dressings could be complemented by more innovative technologies using NPWT. Also in this case, HTA analyses are important to define all the multidimensional advantages. One such analysis was conducted by Nicolazzo and colleagues [17] who linked evidence-based information to real-life practice and expert opinion. In their narrative literature review, a higher efficacy and safety profile emerged for NPWT compared to standard wound care, with the results being also validated by the healthcare professionals who reported that NPWT correlated with a lower rate of occurrence of severe and moderate side effects, leading to significant benefits for patient management. The economic analysis, based on the collection of real-world data, demonstrated that NPWT could optimize the clinical pathway for all patients, with overall savings per patient of 15%, indicating sustainability for the hospital budget. The ability of NPWT to shorten hospital stays and, as a result, free up hospital beds, presents a unique opportunity to improve the patient's clinical pathway while also improving overall access to care. Additionally, NPWT might result in a decrease of social costs related to the patients and caregivers (−28%).

22.4   Health Technology Assessment Within the Setting of Surgical Infections: Strengths and Weaknesses, Opportunities, and Threats

HTA has the potential to improve the management of SSI by providing evidence-based recommendations and promoting cost-effective strategies, also focusing on other important issues such as organizational impact and patient perspectives. In an attempt to summarize the strategic importance of this tool within the SSI setting, a SWOT (strengths, weaknesses, opportunities, and threats) analysis was conducted to define these four aspects as they apply to HTA (Table 22.2).

Table 22.2 SWOT analysis on Health Technology Assessment (HTA) activities conducted within the surgical infections setting

Strengths	Weaknesses
Evidence-based decision-making	*Data limitations*
HTA provides a systematic, evidence-based approach to assess the effectiveness and safety of surgical infection management strategies, enabling healthcare providers and policymakers to make well-informed decisions	HTA requires access to robust data, which may not always be readily available or comprehensive for surgical infection management
Impact on costs	*Time-consuming*
HTA helps identify cost-effective interventions and resource allocation strategies	Conducting an HTA could be time-consuming, which may delay the implementation of necessary changes in clinical practice or healthcare policy
Improved patient outcomes	*Resource-intensive*
By promoting the adoption of best practices and effective interventions, HTA could lead to better patient outcomes and improved quality of care	HTA can be resource-intensive, requiring skilled personnel, data analysis, and financial investment, which may not be feasible in all settings
Interdisciplinary collaboration	*Resistance to change*
HTA typically involves collaboration among healthcare professionals, researchers, economists, and other stakeholders, fostering a holistic approach	Healthcare professionals may resist changes in practice or policies recommended by HTA, especially if they challenge established clinical routines
Opportunities	**Threats**
Innovation adoption	*Resistance from stakeholders*
HTA could facilitate the adoption of innovative technologies and approaches for surgical infection management, leading to improved outcomes and patient safety	Resistance from healthcare professionals, industry stakeholders, or policymakers who may not agree with the findings or recommendations of an HTA can be a significant threat
Global standardization	*Incomplete data*
HTA could help standardize surgical infection management guidelines and practices on a global scale, enhancing consistency in care and reinforce the generalizability of approaches	Inadequate or incomplete data can result in biased or inconclusive HTA findings, potentially leading to incorrect decisions
Healthcare sustainability	*Economic and political pressures*
By identifying cost-effective interventions, HTA could contribute to the sustainability of healthcare systems	Economic constraints and political pressures could influence the outcomes of HTA, potentially compromising the objectivity of the assessment
Patient-centered care	*Lack of standardization*
HTA could prioritize patient-centered care by considering patient-reported outcomes and preferences	Variability in HTA methods and processes across regions or organizations could hinder the comparability of findings and the development of standardized guidelines

References

1. Omachonu VK, Einspruch NG. Innovation in healthcare delivery systems: a conceptual framework. Innov J Public Sect Innov J. 2010;15:2.
2. Bozic KJ, Pierce RG, Herndon JH. Health care technology assessment. Basic principles and clinical applications. J Bone Joint Surg Am. 2004;86(6):1305–14.
3. Scally G, Donaldson LJ. The NHS's 50 anniversary. Clinical governance and the drive for quality improvement in the new NHS in England. BMJ. 1998;317(7150):61–5.
4. Drummond MF, Schwartz JS, Jönsson B, et al. Key principles for the improved conduct of health technology assessments for resource allocation decisions. Int J Technol Assess Health Care. 2008;24(3):244–58; discussion 362–8
5. Kristensen FB. Health technology assessment in Europe. Scand J Public Health. 2009;37(4):335–9.
6. Kumar A, Roberts D, Wood KE, et al. Duration of hypotension before initiation of effective antimicrobial therapy is the critical determinant of survival in human septic shock. Crit Care Med. 2006;34(6):1589–96.
7. Coulter A, Ellins J. Effectiveness of strategies for informing, educating, and involving patients. BMJ. 2007;335(7609):24–7.
8. Badia JM, Casey AL, Petrosillo N, et al. Impact of surgical site infection on healthcare costs and patient outcomes: a systematic review in six European countries. J Hosp Infect. 2017;96(1):1–15.
9. Mujagic E, Marti WR, Coslovsky M, et al. Associations of hospital length of stay with surgical site infections. World J Surg. 2018;42(12):3888–96.
10. Foglia E, Ferrario L, Garagiola E, et al. Economic and organizational sustainability of a negative-pressure portable device for the prevention of surgical-site complications. Clinicoecon Outcomes Res. 2017;9:343–51.
11. Bullough L, Wilkinson D, Burns S, Wan L. Changing wound care protocols to reduce postoperative caesarean section infection and readmission. Wounds UK. 2014;10:72–6.
12. Witt-Majchrzak A, Żelazny P, Snarska J. Preliminary outcome of treatment of postoperative primarily closed sternotomy wounds treated using negative pressure wound therapy. Pol Przegl Chir. 2014;86(10):456–65.
13. Madrid E, Urrútia G, Roqué i Figuls M, et al. Active body surface warming systems for preventing complications caused by inadvertent perioperative hypothermia in adults. Cochrane Database Syst Rev. 2016;4(4):CD009016.
14. Association of periOperative Registered Nurses (AORN). Recommended practices for the prevention of unplanned perioperative hypothermia. In: Perioperative standards and recommended practices. Denver, CO: AORN; 2010. p. 491–504.
15. Sumida H, Sugino S, Kuratani N, et al. Effect of forced-air warming by an underbody blanket on end-of-surgery hypothermia: a propensity score-matched analysis of 5063 patients. BMC Anesthesiol. 2019;19(1):50.
16. Zucconi G, Marchello AM, De Marco C, et al. Health Technology Assessment for the prevention of peri-operative hypothermia: evaluation of the correct use of forced-air warming systems in an Italian hospital. Int J Environ Res Public Health. 2022;20(1):133.
17. Nicolazzo D, Rusin E, Varese A, Galassi M. Negative pressure wound therapy and traditional dressing: an Italian Health Technology Assessment evaluation. Int J Environ Res Public Health. 2023;20(3):2400.

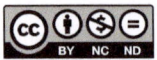